OB-CE1-111

The Vegan Diet As Chronic Disease Prevention

Evidence Supporting the New Four Food Groups

✠

Kerrie K. Saunders,
M.S., L.L.P., C.A.C.-1, C.P.C., Ph.D.

Lantern Books • New York
A Division of Booklight Inc.

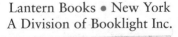

2003
Lantern Books
One Union Square West, Suite 201
New York, NY 10003

Library of Congress Cataloging-in-Publication Data

Saunders, Kerrie.
 The vegan diet as chronic disease prevention : evidence supporting the new four food groups / Kerrie Saunders.
 p. ; cm.
Includes bibliographical references and index.
 ISBN 1-59056-038-8 (alk. paper)
 1. Vegetarianism—Popular works. 2. Diet—in disease—Popular works.
3. Medicine, Preventive—Popular works.
 [DNLM: 1. Chronic Disease—Popular Works. 2. Primary
Prevention—Popular Works. 3. Nutrition Policy—Popular Works. 4.
Vegetarianism—Popular Works. WT 500 S257v 2002] I. Title.
 RM236 .S355 2002
 613.2'62—dc21

printed on 100% post-consumer waste paper, chlorine-free

To Marcella, who shared with me her journey to birth as I finished my dissertation. My thoughts of the pure joy of having her here were the inspiration for its completion.

ACKNOWLEDGMENTS

I AM VERY GRATEFUL FOR THE CONTRIBUTIONS of the following individuals to the person I am today and to the person I am becoming. My mom, Betty, practiced the principles of preventive medicine considered "new breakthroughs" in our home beginning in the early 1960s. My dad, Ray, always seemed to be able to fix anything mechanically wrong in life, and kept me in touch with my conscience and direction through our talks about what was "right." My brother, Rick, is so special to me that my memories of life seem to begin when he was born. I am fortunate to come from a family respectful of the wisdom of God's created nature—a system of systems analogous to the human body, dependent upon proper care for optimal function and longevity. My husband, Mark, encouraged me to pursue my goals and to complete my doctorate, and my wonderful daughter, Marcella, waited so patiently while I revised this text. I am grateful to Lisa, the first vegetarian I met, and to Barry and family, the first vegans I met. I would also like to thank personal friends and family who have supported and loved me, especially John. I also wish to acknowledge the professionals who have inspired me: Richard Knight, D.O.; K. S. Kynell, Ph.D.; Shawn Hatch, M.S.W., C.A.C.; Barbara

Talbot, Ph.D.; John McDougall, M.D.; Neal Barnard, M.D.; Michael Klaper, M.D.; Joel Fuhrman, M.D., Jennifer Raymond, M.S.; Caldwell Esselstyn, M.D.; and especially Michael Greger, M.D. Finally, I am grateful for the wisdom and energy of my editor, Sarah Gallogly.

INFORMATION FOR READERS

✠

THIS BOOK IS MEANT TO SERVE AS A COMPILATION of data supporting the author's view that personal behavioral choices such as diet are the most powerful strategies in maintaining excellent health and in preventing chronic disease. In today's atmosphere of "integrated medicine" (the marriage of chemical, surgical, and technological techniques with natural, organic, and energetic techniques), an individual has the right and the responsibility to research and practice all health-promoting behaviors and attitudes that resonate with his or her soul. In some cases, dietary changes recommended by the experts cited in this book may reduce or eradicate current chronic disease medication needs. These changes should always be made with the assistance and monitoring of one's health care provider. This book is not meant to provide personal advice to individuals without specific knowledge of their unique genetic makeup. There are many important factors in the determination of quantity recommendations for specific nutrients, including age, gender, liver function, and health status; therefore determinations should be made with a competent dietitian or physician. All questions or changes in current approach should be directed to a health care provider who is aware of your individual health status. There is a serious potential risk to sick people who attempt to proceed with treatments in the absence of trained medical supervision, especially when their underlying disease has gone undiagnosed or been treated only in symptom.

CONTENTS

✠

LIST OF TABLES

✢

PREFACE

✣

AMERICA IS ONE OF THE SICKEST NATIONS ON the planet. Despite our wealth, access to educational media, natural resources, and opportunity, most Americans accept atherosclerosis, cancer, hypertension, osteoporosis, heart disease, stroke, diabetes, and other degenerative chronic diseases as a part of the normal aging process. Unfortunately, most "conventional" medical practitioners accept this misguided and bleak picture out of ignorance, though many have expressed a desire to know more about the connection between diet and disease. The Committee on Nutrition in Medical Education (CNME) recommended back in 1985 that a minimum of twenty-five hours would be necessary to teach basic nutrition material, and found that only two medical schools in the nation met these criteria. The CNME also found that less than 3% of the questions on national physician exams for board certification asked about nutrition.[1] By May 2000, medical and osteopathic schools provided an average of only six to thirty hours of nutrition education (including material that was presented outside of nutrition courses).[2] The American Association of Medical Colleges and other accrediting bodies have allowed conditions so lax that some graduating physicians in a traditional curriculum have only received one course in nutrition—the safest, most effective and inexpensive form of chronic disease prevention available. Worse yet, this one course is guided by the United States Department of Agriculture (USDA) Food Pyramid of 1992, and was previously based upon the Basic Four Food Groups of 1956. These faulty and dangerous dietary guidelines gained and retain their place thanks to heavy lobbying by the meat and dairy industries, whose political dollars find their way to the individual pockets or the campaign funds of officials in Washington, D.C. In 1988, the United States Surgeon General announced that about two thirds of all deaths in America were related to diet.[3] This book will compile scientific evidence and prove beyond reasonable doubt that our Standard American Diet (SAD) keeps Americans sick—and makes others sick who switch to it.

Using current technology and data spanning thousands of years, gathered from paleopathologists and other scientific researchers around the world, the Physicians' Committee for Responsible Medicine (PCRM) and others have compared cultural dietary practices and resultant chronic disease incidence rates. This is precisely the work that our government should have done decades ago with our tax dollars. Instead, the United States Government, the American Medical Association (AMA), and the American Dietetic Association (ADA) have shown us through their actions that they are controlled by the livestock, dairy, and other lobbies and are willing to compromise human lives and squander taxpayer dollars. In light of the evidence, I see no other explanation.

Between 1970 and 1986, Americans watched the amount of money spent annually on legal drugs rise from $8 billion to $31 billion. During this same time period, the total disease care bill for Americans rose from 7.4% to 11% of the nation's Gross National Product.[4] The current trend shows the picture worsening exponentially while Americans become sick and watch their loved ones die painful deaths. As Dr. John McDougall has said, the current American health care system would be more appropriately called an "illness-care system."[5]

In the following pages, I will summarize existing research on various dietary practices and their subsequent preventable disease incidence rates. I will also introduce the vegan New Four Food Groups and focus upon specific and commonly occurring preventable diseases related to the Standard American Diet (SAD). Finally, I'll discuss related ethical and political issues, along with positive trends and what they indicate about our food choices today. In the appendices, physicians and their patients will find educational fact sheets that they can photocopy and distribute freely.

D.W. Cavanaugh, M.D., of Cornell University, wrote, "There is only one major disease and that is malnutrition. All ailments and afflictions to which we may fall heir are directly traceable to this major disease."[6] If these statements sound radical to you now, I invite you to read further and form your own judgment.

---

1.   National Academy of Sciences, *Nutrition Education in U.S. Medical Schools* (Washington, D.C.: National Academy Press, 1985), cited in J. S. Novick, "Effects of a Nutrition Education Program on the Related Knowledge and

Behaviors of Family Practice Residents" (master's thesis, Indiana State University, 2000, 2001).

2. Torti Jr., Frank M., et al. "Survey of Nutrition Education in U.S. Medical Schools: An Instructor-Based Analysis" (*Medical Education Online*, 2001).

3. Koop, C. Everett, and the United States Department of Health and Human Services, Public Health Service, *The Surgeon General's Report on Nutrition and Health* (California: Prima Publishing, 1988, and New York: St. Martin's Press, July 1988).

4. Jensen, Bernard, M.D., and Mark Anderson, *Empty Harvest: Understanding the Link between Our Food, Our Immunity, and Our Planet* (New York: Avery Publishing, 1990), 114–115.

5. McDougall, John A., M.D., *McDougall's Medicine: A Challenging Second Opinion* (Clinton, NJ: New Win Publishing, Inc., 1985), 13.

6. Quoted in Jensen, op. cit.

1

HISTORICAL COMPARISONS
OF DIETARY PRACTICES
AND RESULTANT DISEASE PREVALENCE

HOMO SAPIENS APPEARED APPROXIMATELY 40,000 years ago, and we have evidence of agricultural practices beginning about 10,000 years ago. Since that time, the human diet remained virtually unchanged until a little over 100 years ago, when the Industrial Revolution drastically changed both our food supply and our activity level.[1] Organic and nutrient-rich natural foods grown in a perfect ecosystem with clean, fresh air and water have now been replaced by "technologically advanced" but nutrient-stripped versions, laced with nonbiodegradable synthetic chemicals, antibiotics, and hormones. In addition, the human dietary intake of animals has increased dramatically. The result has been weakened human bodies with an incidence rate of 80–90% or more of death by diseases—such as cancer, cardiovascular disease, stroke, and diabetes—caused by diet.

Current studies of traditional human dietary practices challenge the idea that humans were aggressive hunting animals who depended primarily on animal flesh for survival. According to the research, the prehistoric diet for at least the last million and a half years was primarily three times more plant than animal foods,[2] the reverse of what the average

American eats on the Standard American Diet (referred to from here onward as the SAD).

Paleopathologists (scientists who study mummies, frozen skeletons, and other remains) can now tell us which chronic diseases were and were not present in humans at different times, and have drawn conclusions regarding dietary influences. From paleopathology, we have learned that cultures with primarily animal-centered diets, such as the meat-eating nobility of recent centuries, suffered many of the same diseases that we do today, including heart disease, hardening of the arteries, cancer, gallstones, kidney stones, osteoporosis, arthritis, tooth decay, gout, and even headaches. Interestingly, these diseases were *not* present in humans eating plant-based diets, e.g., most of the primitive human cultures, and the peasants, slaves, and "common folk" of recent human history. Their diet has been proven to consist mainly of apples, barley, leeks, garlic, lentils, melons, onions, radishes, seeds, wheat, and other plant foods. Some ancient societies ate more animal foods, but the amount and type of fat consumed was very different from what it is today. Modern domesticated farm animals contain about eight to ten times more fat than their wild counterparts.[3] The European nobility of the last few centuries ate mainly the flesh of cows, goats, sheep, ducks, and geese, and their remains show evidence of all of the diseases that are now attributed to the consumption of animal proteins and fats.[4]

Some people believe the myth that Americans are living longer and are much healthier than they were in the past. In fact, the life expectancy for a 45-year-old increased by only six years from 1870 to 1970, despite sterile hospitals, improved sanitation, technological advances, and the invention of vaccines and antibiotics that protect us from cholera, typhoid, chicken pox, yellow fever, bubonic plague, tuberculosis, and most venereal diseases. Some statisticians will cite figures that appear to indicate better medical progress in life expectancy, but these often do not factor out infant mortality (which was fifteen times higher in 1870 than in 1970) and maternal birthing mortality rates. The obvious major change that occurred within those 100 years is that Americans began to eat very differently than they had in the past.[5] Therefore, although antibiotics and other advances have helped with many ills, we now die of atherosclerosis, obesity, cancer, diabetes, and other chronic diseases that can be prevented perhaps 80–90% of the time by proper nutritional habits.

As the following references will show, the understanding that proper diet has a key role in good health is not a new one. On the contrary, all of the world's major religions and cultures recognize the life-sustaining or life-destroying abilities of diet.

Many readers will be familiar with the biblical story of Daniel, and may remember the dietary experiment described therein. After suffering with ill health, Daniel proposed switching the servants from the rich "royal" foods to a diet of vegetables and water. In only ten days' time, the servants looked healthier and better nourished than any of the young men who had eaten the "royal" foods (Daniel 1:11–15).

We can trace other dietary recommendations to the Bible, which outlines what is now called the kosher diet. "God said, 'See, I give you all the seed-bearing plants that are upon the whole earth, and all the trees with seed-bearing fruit; this

shall be your food' " (Genesis 1:29). "The Lord spoke to
Moses, saying: 'Speak to the sons of Israel, say to them: "You
must not eat the fat of ox, sheep or goat. The fat of an animal that has died a natural death or been savaged by beasts
may be used for any other purpose, but you must not eat it"
' " (Leviticus 7:23–24). The diet later allowed the eating of
specific animals (which, unlike the animals most Americans
eat today, were devoid of synthetic hormones, pesticides, herbicides, and antibiotics). The text specifically forbids the eating of camel, hyrax, hare, pig, and any sea life that is without fins or scales: "You must hold them detestable; you are
not to eat their flesh and you must avoid their carcasses"
(Leviticus 11:1–12). Scales or not, keep in mind how many
more toxins are present in our planet's waters at this date,
nearly 4,000 years later.

"You must not eat any of the following birds: eagles,
owls, hawks, falcons, buzzards, vultures, crows, ostriches,
seagulls, storks, herons, pelicans, cormorants, hoopoes, or
bats" (Leviticus 11:9–13). We now have scientifically established that these animals are dangerous to eat—shellfish, for
example, with their high concentrations of mercury, contaminants, and toxins; and the scavenger birds and animals who
carry diseases such as rabies, tuberculosis, trichinosis, salmonella, and parasites.

Further, in keeping with current studies of the excreted
waste products and other contaminants found in animal and
human blood (ureas, bilirubin, creatinine, creatine, uric acid,
organic acids, ketoglutaric acid, malic acid, hormones, pyru-
vic acid, lipids, cholesterol, etc.), the Bible says, "It shall be a
perpetual statute throughout your generations, in all your

dwelling places, that you eat neither fat nor blood" (Leviticus 3:17). "Moreover you shall eat no blood whatever, whether of fowl or of animal, in any of your dwellings" (Leviticus 7:25–26).

Here is just a sampling of both ancient and modern dietary recommendations from around the world:

- One of the world's oldest medical books, the *Yellow Emperor's Classic of Internal Medicine* or *Nei Ching,* was written in the third century B.C.E., or possibly much earlier. It recommends whole cereal grains as the principal food. *Ching*'s followers were said to have lived actively until over 100 years of age.

- The *Upanishads*, also called the early Forest Teachings of India, state, "From food are born all creatures; they live upon food, they are dissolved in food. Food is the chief of all things, the universal medicine."

- The principal texts of Ayurveda emphasize the central importance of dietary intake in health: "[T]he use of food that is injurious is the cause of disease."

- The Quran teaches of the beneficial effects of grains, as did the twelfth-century Jewish physician and philosopher Moses Maimonides.

- The medieval medical system taught by Ibn Sina (Avicenna), long the standard in Europe and the Middle East, placed the importance of a healthy diet at the center of its medical teachings.

- In 1713, the renowned Japanese physician and Confucian scholar Ekiken Kaibara, who remains a prominent force in Japanese medicine, recommended a balanced diet and light, simple meals as protection against chronic disease.

- In the eighteenth century, Christophe Von Hufeland, Goethe's physician, wrote on macrobiotics and warned of the health hazards of meat and sugar.

- Eighteenth-century Japanese physiognomist Namboku Mizuno recommended a simple grain and vegetable diet. "But someone who loves sake, meat, and rich food," he said, "will spoil his mind and body, and automatically he will destroy such great 'ki' energy, and his life will be short."

- Japanese physician Sagen Ishizuka concluded at the end of the nineteenth century, from studies in anthropology and the military, that the ideal diet is based on whole cereal grains supplemented by beans, vegetables, seeds, and nuts, with a small amount of fish or game depending on the climate, region, and season.

- Dr. Albert Schweitzer, who spent over forty years working in French equatorial Africa, attributed the rise of degenerative disease to the import of European foods, such as condensed milk, canned butter, meat and fish preserves, white bread, and refined salt.

- In 1913, George Ohsawa (also called Yukikazu Sakurazawa) healed himself of terminal pulmonary tuberculosis with health and diet recommendations by Sagen Ishikuza, and then spent over fifty years teaching macrobiotic methods of eating.[6]

- John Stuart, an English traveler across Europe and Asia and an observer of many cultures, said, "I have observed among nations whose aliment is vegetables and water that disease and medicine are equally unknown, while those whose aliment is flesh and fermented liquor are constantly afflicted with disease and with medicine more dangerous than disease itself."[7]

- Finally, almost 2,500 years ago, studying in ancient Greece, Hippocrates—also called the "Father of Medicine"—stated, "Let food be thy medicine and thy medicine food." Interestingly, medical schools have edited out the reference to diet from the original Hippocratic Oath, which stated, "I will apply dietetic measures for the benefit of the sick according to my ability and judgment; I will keep them from harm and injustice." Hippocrates recommended a diet rich in plant-based foods native to their environment.[8]

The health statistics yielded by current scientific studies on various existing cultures are also of interest. The Tarahumara and Hunza cultures, for example, are receiving great attention due to their excellent health.

The Mexican Tarahumara Indians in the Sierra Madre Occidental Mountains eat a diet that is roughly equivalent to the Pritikin Diet (10% protein, 10% fat, and 80% carbohydrates). Research cited in recent years noted that their cholesterol levels average 125 mg/dl, compared to the average American Caucasian at 220–280 mg/dl.[9] On this diet, the Tarahumaras can perform a 500-mile run in five days and carry a 100-pound pack for 110 miles in 70 hours. It has been noted that the women of the tribe can run continuously for 50 miles at a time. These Indians eat animal protein perhaps once a month; their main diet consists of corn, peas, beans, squash, and other native plants and fruits. Physical examinations show that they are completely free from cardiovascular disease, hypertension, diabetes, and obesity.[10] The 50,000 Tarahumaras use no mechanical energy in farming and travel only by foot.[11]

The people living in Pakistan's Hunza Valley eat almost exclusively home-grown, organic plant foods, such as fruits, grains, and vegetables, fed by glacial mineral water. The main Hunza grain is millet, and they never consume bleached, enriched, processed foods. The Hunza people eat animal protein very infrequently, and their health is unrivaled anywhere in the world. Not only do they have no chronic disease and no need for hospitals, dentists, or doctors, but they also seem to have no need for police, army, prisons, and mental health institutions. Individuals over 100 years old still have smooth skin, clear eyes, and all of their teeth.[12]

Robert McCarrison, a British surgeon, traveled through the Northwest Territory of India for seven years, from 1904 to 1911, and studied the Hunza there. He stated, "I never saw a case of asthenic dyspepsia, of gastric or duodenal ulcer, of appendicitis, of mucous colitis, or of cancer."[13]

Shifts from traditional plant-based diets to animal-based diets have also been proven to cause diseases like diabetes among the Pima Native American Indians; the Yemenites, who moved to Israel and changed their diet; and Kurdish immigrants.[14]

The U.S. government didn't have most of this information in the late 1800s and early to mid-1900s, at the time of the large American demographic shift from country to city, when its regulation of foods began to focus on convenience rather than nutritional value. America's food supply became homogenized, pasteurized, refined, bleached, chemically preserved, hydrogenized, defibered, artificially flavored and colored, synthetically fortified, sugared, and salted. (Today, plants and animals are also genetically engineered, irradiated, antibiotic-fed, and laden with pesticides, herbicides, and hormones.) Just as the doctors who used to recommend smoking to their "nervous" patients or white sugar to their overweight patients[15] didn't know how mistaken these ideas were, our government was probably unaware of the dangers of allowing animal products and re-packaged "convenience" foods to replace whole fruits, grains, and vegetables.

But now, despite the substantial evidence against the SAD and in support of a vegan diet, our government continues to perpetuate debilitating, expensive, and painful disease for millions of Americans through its purposely lackadaisical regulation of the curriculums of the American Medical Association (AMA) and the American Dietetic Association (ADA). Dr. Albert Stunkard states, "Failures of nutrition education do not stop at the elementary school level. The poor state of nutrition education in higher education, notably in medical school, is undoubtedly one of the many factors contributing to the nutrition problem—including obesity—of our nation."[16] Until Americans demand more from their government, and from their physicians and other medical leaders, our country will remain sick and tired for unfortunate generations to come. We must demand it with our refusal to intellectually and financially support any compromise of proven disease prevention based on statistical comparisons that are already available. We do not need to await further experimentally controlled conditions, bureaucratic funding, or support from the AMA or the ADA.

The meat and dairy industries have such a tight hold on the U.S. government's Department of Agriculture that they successfully delayed the release of the "Food Pyramid" for a full year, asking the Department of Agriculture to reconsider its graphic design wherein meat and dairy were portrayed close to the top, near "Fats, Oils, and Sweets."[17] As you read on, consider what that one year meant in terms of millions of lives lost and billions of dollars wasted as the "Basic Four Food Groups" remained in place as America's guide to optimum health. This situation is good business for the meat and dairy industries and their elected officials, but terrible business for taxpayers when we look at the cost in human lives, governmental assistance benefits, hospital and medical costs, time off work due to disease and disability, and health education dollars wasted on programs that can have little if any positive effect on current disease statistics if used "as directed" by consumers.

It is the author's opinion that, just as the "Basic Four Food Groups" of the 1950s (which instructed us to be sure to eat four or more servings of whole milk products each day, along with the equivalent of 12 ounces of red meat) are now known to be misguided, so will the Food Pyramid become obsolete to the generations that follow ours. It is the author's hope that the Food Pyramid will be replaced—before another 40-year waiting period has passed—by the vegan "New

Four Food Groups" as a guideline with which to educate our citizens and our children.

Many nations have noted the human and financial costs of poor dietary practices and have responded with new policies, though some of these still represent compromised, not faithful, adherence to the facts.

Dietary goals for the United Kingdom were summarized in Britain's foremost medical journal, the *Lancet*, after the National Advisory Committee on Nutritional Education (NACNE) issued conclusions in its 1983 report. The Committee had studied British dietary trends over time, and was able to justify its conclusions based on longitudinal research observation. The report called for an increase in fiber intake, and for reductions in fat, sugar, salt, and alcohol. Reductions were also called for in specifically mentioned foods that had been added to the British diet since 1945, including highly processed foods and items that "are not British in origin (e.g., hamburgers, yogurt, pasta)."[18]

Interestingly, as Japan became "westernized," importing American-style foods, restaurants, and rushed eating habits, its health became "westernized," too. Japan's fat consumption jumped from less than 10% calories from fat in 1955 to 25% calories from fat in 1987.[19] In 1985, the Japanese Ministry of Health and Welfare issued dietary recommendations that included the reduction of total fat, saturated fat, and salt. The Ministry encouraged people to adopt a varied diet, increase home cooking and use of vegetable and fish oil, and to create a pleasant eating environment.[20] Epidemiologists reported that cancer of the lung, breast, and colon increased two to three times among Japanese women between 1950 and

1975. During this period, cow milk consumption increased fifteen times; meat, chicken egg, and poultry consumption increased over seven times; and rice consumption dropped 70%.[21] Scientists have also observed that coronary heart disease rates tripled (in one generation) in Japanese who migrated to the West Coast of the United States, and doubled among Japanese who migrated to Hawaii.[22] These data undermine previously existing theories of a genetic superiority in the health of the Japanese culture; i.e., when their diet changed, their health status changed as well.

Rastafari, a movement no longer confined to Jamaica, where it originated, is gaining in popularity.[23] Often considered in the past to be a community of "dreadlocked" hairstyles, reggae music, and marijuana smokers, Rastafari has evolved into a multicultural movement of spiritual principles that espouses a vegan diet, exercise and massage routines, and abstention from caffeine, salt, and canned or preserved foods.

Many of our ancestors left old-world Europe, with its monarchies and class systems, in search of life, liberty, and the pursuit of happiness. In the environment from which they came, the aristocrats and royalty had modeled a "rich" diet of animal flesh and dairy products. Denied these foods by lack of wealth, our forebears mistakenly pursued them and associated them emotionally with the attainment of "the good life." Unfortunately, this new diet now affords us all of the discomforts that plagued the wealthy European aristocrats and royalty of old: gout, arthritis, diabetes, obesity, etc. Images come to mind of the overweight kings and queens who had to be carried everywhere due to their obesity, related inactivity, fatigue, and disease.

We often take pride in being taller than our ancestors, and have been told that our increased stature is a result of eating more protein than previous generations. But I propose that we are slightly taller because of the natural and synthetic growth hormones present in the animal flesh and fluids that provide that extra protein in our diet—and because of the refined sugars (which can have a stimulant effect on the body and disrupt metabolism) in the packaged foods we eat today. As I will demonstrate in later chapters, these factors, on their own or in combination, have contributed to an increase not only in height, but also in obesity, breast cancer, early onset of menstruation, and deadly atherosclerotic complications such as heart attack and stroke. Some of the ramifications of this will be discussed further in later chapters.

In 1977, the McGovern Senate Select Committee on Nutrition and Human Needs Report recommended a reduction in the American diet from 42% calories from fat to 30%.[24] This came after two years of public hearings with vegetarian and macrobiotic teachers, nutritionists, schoolteachers, corrections officials, parents, and other concerned citizens. Until this time, the government and much of the scientific and medical community had been basically silent about the typical SAD—high in meat and other animal products, sugar, refined flour, highly processed foods, and foods grown or treated with chemicals, additives, and other artificial ingredients. The Report helped to expose the link between the modern diet and six of the leading causes of death in the U.S., including heart disease and cancer.[25]

Nationally recognized surveys like the Nationwide Food Consumption Survey and the National Health and Nutrition

Survey indicate that average American fat consumption is actually between 37% and 38% calories,[26] while the planet's healthy cultures eat a diet that is closer to 10–15% calories from fat. Our increased consumption of fat and decreased consumption of complex carbohydrates in the last 150 years or so has been implicated as the main causative factor in increased mortality from heart disease in many cross-referenced international studies. One of these studies, in which the Harvard School of Public Health compared three groups of men (Irish men living in Ireland, their brothers who had emigrated to Boston, and unrelated men of Irish descent living in Boston), concluded further that fiber intake and vegetable consumption were lower among the men who died from coronary artery disease.[27]

Many of the authorities cited within this book are not only highly credentialed and educated but are also testimonial case histories. For example, Nathan Pritikin was diagnosed with hypercholesterolemia, atherosclerosis, and posterior wall myocardial ischemia. Pritikin states that he lowered his own cholesterol count from 300 to 120 through a vegan diet (similar to his marketed diet plan, in which, however, animal products are basically used as "condiments"), and received a normal electrocardiogram—the beginnings of restored excellent health.[28]

Another example is Dr. John McDougall, who, as a young man, suffered a stroke accompanied by paralysis that lasted for several months. Later, as a physician, he grew disappointed with the medical profession's inability to prevent and treat the recurrence of chronic illnesses such as his. He estimates that 85% of the patients in hospitals today are suffering from symptoms associated with diet-induced diseases, such as obesity, heart disease, hypertension, stroke, diabetes, and cancer. While traditional medicine has made incredible leaps in the diagnostic, acute trauma, rehabilitation, and surgical areas, it has largely failed to address the prevention of chronic disease.

Dr. McDougall began the process of educating himself in the role of nutrition and diet in human health, a subject ignored in most medical curriculums. He also made changes in his family's diet at home. He describes first eliminating red meat, then all animal flesh, then dairy products, and finally oils in *The New McDougall Cookbook*. He follows the family's transformation from "sickly carnivores to healthy vegetarians" noting their increased energy, the disappearance of constipation, stomachaches, and oily skin, and the loss of excess weight—as well as a significant drop in his own blood cholesterol level.

Dr. McDougall also observed these transformations in his patients as they made similar dietary changes. He recalls confrontations with superiors during the early years of his medical practice. One medical supervisor even suggested to him that it might be tough for a physician to make a living without patients needing to return for continuous prescription refills.[29]

In Table 1, Dr. McDougall offers a list of diseases for which a "rich" western diet is a *primary causative factor*. A primary causative factor is an element that must be present in order for a disease to develop. Diet is a controllable primary factor, like smoking, alcohol use, lack of exercise, and improper stress management. Genetic predisposition is an

TABLE 1.		
DISEASES CAUSED BY A "RICH" WESTERN DIET		
Systemic Diseases	Bowel Disorders	Cancers
Allergies	Appendicitis	Breast
Arthritis	Colitis	Colon
Atherosclerosis	Constipation	Kidney
Adult diabetes	Diarrhea	Pancreas
Gout	Diverticulosis	Prostate
Heart attacks	Gallstones	Testicle
Hormone imbalance	Gastritis	Uterus (body)
Hypertension	Hemorrhoids	
Kidney failure	Hiatus hernia	
Kidney stones	Indigestion	
Multiple sclerosis	Malabsorption	
Obesity	Polyps	
Osteoporosis	Ulcers	
Strokes		

Reprinted from McDougall, John A., M.D., *The McDougall Program* (New York: Penguin Group, 1990), 5 by permission of John A. McDougall, M.D.

uncontrollable factor. Secondary factors only aggravate the existing disease process.

The vegan New Four Food Groups not only allow us to live free of many of these chronic diseases (as you will read in later chapters of this book), but also offer other undeniable health benefits. Some brief examples from the scientific literature include:

- Twenty-five patients with bronchial asthma were put on a vegan diet, and showed a 71% improvement within four months and a 92% improvement after one year.[30]

- Investigators at Wayne State University found 100% improvement in patients suffering from rheumatoid arthritis when they ate a fat-free diet (also naturally lower in reactive food antigens) for only six weeks. The symptoms recurred within 72 hours of the reintroduction of vegetable oil or animal fat into the diet. The researchers concluded that dietary fat in the amounts normally eaten in the American diet cause inflammatory joint changes seen in rheumatoid arthritis.[31]

- The vegan diet has been shown to improve Swedish patients suffering from rheumatoid arthritis.[32]

- The Farm, a large vegan community in Tennessee, was the source of a study on 1,700 pregnancies and their outcomes. Only 1 in 100 were delivered by cesarean section, compared to 1 in 4 currently in America's general population. Further, in 20 years, only one case of preeclampsia was found in the 1,700 pregnancies, compared to 2 in 100 in America's general population.[33]

While most of the modern medical community continues to ignore the mounting evidence, awareness of the consequences of poor dietary habits is spreading among the general public. Agatha Thrash, M.D., wrote a warning in 1998 that still holds true today: "Our country is filled with people who are sick or disabled from the excess of nutrients they are taking. The excess is almost always in the direction of specific nutrient excesses, such as too much fat or refined car-bohydrates. Degenerative diseases follow these specific excesses. It is now possible to predict which types of diseases a population will suffer from by studying the pattern of its nutritive excesses and deficiencies. Excesses in fats lead to heart and artery disease, malignancies, hepatic and digestive diseases. Excesses in refined carbohydrates lead to metabolic diseases such as diabetes, the 'Hypoglycemic syndrome' and stress-related diseases, liver and pancreatic disorders, neuro-logic and psychiatric conditions."[34]

As we begin to see disease as an injury or an imbalance at its molecular level, we can begin to understand the pow-erful role of nutrients as strategic weapons of defense—capa-ble of initiating and maintaining health, while combating even the earliest warning signs of danger. When we see food as chemistry in the body, we begin to see the wisdom of a plant-based diet—rich in fiber, enzymes, water, vitamins, minerals, antioxidants and other phytonutrients, with an ideal balance of plant protein. The following chapters will prove the benefit of choosing this diet over one based upon animal flesh and fluids—high in cholesterol and saturated fat, containing many proteins implicated in food allergies and other disorders, and frequently harboring concentrated pesticide and herbicide residues and veterinary hormones and antibiotics. The educated consumer or health care profes-sional, rather than falling victim to marketing tactics, choos-es to see food as chemistry—and shops and eats accordingly.

1. Pawlak, Laura, Ph.D., R.D., *A Perfect 10: Phyto "New-trients" against Cancers,* (Emeryville, CA: Biomed General Corporation, 1998), 1.

2. Brody, Jane E., "Research Yields Surprises About Early Human Diets," *New York Times* science section, May 15, 1979.

3. Eaton, S. B., and Konner, M., "Paleolithic nutrition," *New England Journal of Medicine* 313: 283–289, 1995.

4. Edmonds, Brian, *The Doctors' Book of Bible Healing Foods* (Boca Raton, Florida: Globe Communications Corp., 1992), 5.

5. McDougall, John A., M.D., *The McDougall Program* (New York: Penguin Group, 1990), 53–54.

6. Jack, Alex, *Let Food Be Thy Medicine* (Becket, MA: One Peaceful World Press, 1991), 12–20.

7. Ibid., 17–18.

8. Ibid., 7.

9. *New England Journal of Medicine* (1975), American Heart Association (1980), *American Journal of Medicine* (1986), and the China Health Study (1990), cited in Jack, op. cit., p. 43.

10. Pritikin, Nathan, and Patrick McGrady, *The Pritikin Program for Diet and Exercise* (New York: Grosset and Dunlap, Inc., 1979), 28–29.

11. Jack, *Let Food Be Thy Medicine*, 23.

12. Jensen, Bernard, M.D., and Mark Anderson, *Empty Harvest: Understanding the Link Between Our Food, Our Immunity, and Our Planet* (New York: Avery Publishing, 1990), 159.

13. McCarrison, Robert, M.D., "Faulty food in relation to gastro-intestinal disorder," *Journal of the American Medical Association* 1922; 78: 1–8, cited in Jack, op. cit., 18–19.

14. Cowen, R., "Seeds of Protection," *Science News* 1990; 137: 350–351; Brody, Jane, "Arizona Indians Reclaim Ancient Foods," *New York Times*, May 21, 1991; and Cohen, A. M., "Effect of change in environment on the prevalence of diabetes among Yemenite and Kurdish communities," *Israel Medical Journal* 1960; 19: 137–142, cited in Jack, *Let Food Be Thy Medicine*, 72–73.

15. Jensen, op. cit., 37–40.

16. Stunkard, A. J., "Obesity and the social environment: current status, future prospects," in G. A. Bray, ed., *Obesity in America,* NIH publication #80-359, 1980.

17. Barnard, Neal, M.D., *Food for Life* (New York: Three Rivers Press, 1993), 294.

18. "Implementing the N.A.C.N.E. Report," *Lancet* 1983; 2: 1151–1156, cited in Jack, *Let Food Be Thy Medicine*, 33–34.

19. Wynder, E. L., Fujita, Y., Harris, R. E., Hirayama, T., and Hiyama, T., "Comparative epidemiology of cancer between the United States and Japan," *Cancer*, 1991; 67: 746–763.

20. Panel on Nutrition and Prevention of Diseases, 1983, and *Dietary Guidelines for Health Promotion*, Vol. 29 (Health Promotion and Nutrition Division, Health Services Bureau, Japanese Ministry of Health and Welfare, Tokyo, 1985), cited in Jack, *Let Food Be Thy Medicine*, 34–35.

21. Kagawa, Y., "Impact of Westernization on the nutrition of Japanese: changes in physique, cancer, longevity, and centenarians," *Preventive Medicine*, 1978; 7: 205–217

22. Robertson, T. L., et al., "Epidemiologic Studies of Coronary Heart Disease and Stroke in Japanese Men Living in Japan, Hawaii, and California," *American Journal of Cardiology* 1977; 39: 239–243.

23. Talvi, Silja J. A., "The Ital Life," in *Veggie Life* magazine, July 1998, 45–47.

24. Pritikin, *The Pritikin Program*, xxv.

25. Jack, *Let Food Be Thy Medicine*, 25.

26. Raymond, Jennifer, M.S., "Caution: Approaching the Zone," excerpts cited in *Vegan Outreach* newsletter, June 1, 1998, 9.

27. Kushi, L. H., et al., "Diet and 20-year mortality from coronary heart disease. The Ireland-Boston Diet-Heart Study," *New England Journal of Medicine*, 1985; 312: 811–818.

28. Pritikin, *The Pritikin Program*, 90–93.

29. McDougall, *The McDougall Program*, 16–28.

30. Lindahl, O., et al., "Vegan diet regimen with reduced medication in the treatment of bronchial asthma," *Journal of Asthma* 1985; 22: 45–55.

31. Lucas, P., "Dietary fat aggravates active rheumatoid arthritis," *Clinical Research* 1981; 29: 754A.

32. Skoldstam, L., "Fasting and vegan diet in rheumatoid arthritis," *Scandinavian Journal of Rheumatology* 1987; 15(2): 219–221.

33. Barnard, *Food for Life*, 158.

34. Thrash, Agatha, M.D., *Eat for Strength: A Vegetarian Cookbook, Oil-Free*, (Alabama: Thrash Publications, 1978), 27.

2

THE VEGAN DIET

THE VEGAN "NEW FOUR FOOD GROUPS DIET" AS referenced in this book has been promoted by the Physicians Committee for Responsible Medicine (PCRM), in Washington, D.C., since April 8, 1991.[1] This group represents doctors, nurses, dietitians, researchers, and other concerned citizens who are successfully working toward dietary prevention of America's chronic diseases, and its membership has grown to approximately 10,000. PRCM offers lectures, programs on nutrition education for schools, hospitals, and businesses, a quarterly newsletter, and other services. PCRM states that, based on undeniable scientific evidence, "The typical Western diet, high in animal fat and protein and lacking in fiber, is associated with increased risk of cancer, heart disease, obesity, diabetes, and osteoporosis."[2]

As the reader will observe, many other organizations—such as the American Heart Association, the American Dietetic Association, the Arthritis Foundation, and others receiving funds from politically charged sources—are incestuously tied to the U.S. government (which is heavily lobbied by big business interests like the meat and dairy industries) and will offer compromised and weak health recommendations for the layperson. PCRM, however, has studied research from all over the world, and makes sound recommendations based on all of the data. It is now up to the individual to decide how well he or she would like to function and feel, and to make choices accordingly.

In order to best describe the parameters of the vegan New Four Food Groups, it will be practical to begin with terms that identify the different diets found in nature.

- The **omnivorous** diet includes plants, plant products, animal flesh, animal products, and waste. Omnivores typically have very sharp nails and teeth. Examples include the raccoon, the bear, and the rat.
- The **carnivorous** diet consists almost exclusively of animal flesh and other parts of animals. Carnivores have claws, short intestines, and teeth (or fangs) sharp enough to tear raw flesh from the bone. They pant to cool their bodies, lap water when they drink, and have an unlimited capacity to excrete cholesterol. Examples include the wolf, the tiger, and the lion.
- The **herbivorous** diet consists exclusively of plants and plant products. Herbivores have hands or hooves, long intestines, and flat teeth for grinding fruits, vegetables, and grains. They sweat to cool their bodies, sip water when they drink, and can excrete only very small amounts of cholesterol from their bodies. Examples include the deer, the elephant, the giraffe, the gorilla, and the human.

Although there are indications that the human body has adapted, mutated, or evolved to be able to tolerate small amounts of animal protein, animal-derived iron, and insects, these substances are not required in the design of a healthful human diet.

Further, a brief note is necessary to explain the different "vegetarian" diets chosen by humans:

- The **vegan or pure vegetarian** diet consists of plants and plant products only. It is free of the eggs, flesh, and fluids of animals, including birds, fish, and insects. The New Four Food Groups of the Physicians Committee for Responsible Medicine and the diets espoused by John McDougall, M.D., Joel Fuhrman, M.D., William Harris, M.D., Dean Ornish, M.D., the Pritikin Center, and many others are all vegan or near-vegan diets.
- The **lacto-vegetarian** diet consists of plants, plant products, and the milk or milk products of cows or goats.
- The **ovo-vegetarian** diet consists of plants, plant products, and poultry or fish eggs.
- The **lacto-ovo vegetarian** diet consists of plants, plant products, cow or goat milk or milk products, and poultry or fish eggs.

There are still other popular terms, such as the pesco- or pesce-vegetarian (one who consumes a plant-based diet with the addition of fish), or the pollo-vegetarian (one who consumes a plant-based diet with the addition of chicken), but neither of these cases fits the true definition of a vegetarian, one who abstains from flesh.

While it is unrealistic to expect every person to become a dietitian or to consider in turn the Recommended Dietary Allowance (RDA), the Daily Value (DV), the Reference Daily Intake (RDI), the Daily Reference Value (DRV), and the Upper Limit (UL) of every nutrient in planning a meal, it is not unrealistic to expect to be able to show someone the New Four Food Groups and quickly effect a transition to a more healthful, plant-based diet.

Americans who eat the animal-based SAD would plan a meal centered around a piece of animal flesh (cow, chicken, turkey, tuna, etc.) with an added vegetable or potato, most often swimming in cow-milk butter or cheese. A person eating a vegan diet would plan a meal by selecting a complex carbohydrate starch (rice, corn, quinoa, cereal, lentils, beans, etc.), and then add fruits, vegetables, bread, beans, or pasta to the dish. The four main food groupings in the vegan diet, as recommended by PCRM,[3] are:

Fruits	3 or more servings per day
Grains	5 or more servings per day
Vegetables	3 or more servings per day
Legumes	2 or more servings per day

At first glance, most Americans would agree that all seems to be in order—but they would also notice immediately the absence of meat (animal flesh), eggs, and dairy products (bovine mammary secretions). Meat and dairy industry advertisements have conditioned Americans to see these items as necessary and healthy in a human diet. Popular misconceptions include: "You have to eat meat to get protein," "Starches are all fattening," and "You have to eat cow-milk products for calcium." On the contrary, many of the healthiest populations on the planet exclude animals and animal products from their diets, or eat them so rarely (i.e. in semi-annual ceremonies, during drought or famine, etc.), that they have no observable effect upon their health.

Traditionally educated dietitians, nurses, and physicians are often suspicious of the vegan diet's ability to provide adequate protein, amino acids, calcium, iron, folic acid, and vitamins B12 and D. These specific nutrients will be discussed in detail below.

• PROTEIN

Proteins provide the raw material for many of the functional and structural components of the body. The human body does not need to eat another animal's muscle in order to build its own muscle. Neither do other natural vegetarians, like deer, gorillas, bulls, stallions, giraffes, and elephants.

While there are variations in outcome on vegetarian endurance tests found in scientific literature, probably due to subjective differences in the intake of refined foods, it is interesting to note just a few of the findings over the years regarding the excellent athletic functioning possible on a healthy plant-based diet. In 1907, the *Yale Medical Journal* published findings showing that both vegetarian athletes *and vegetarian non-athletes* excelled in exercise endurance over meat-eating athletes.[4] In 1968, *Nutrition Today* cited a study from Denmark in which researchers found that a high-protein diet rich in cow milk, meat, and chicken eggs slowed energy output on a stationary bike to 57 minutes, but that the same men, on a diet of whole grain cereals, bread, vegetables, and fruit, increased their mean endurance to 2 hours and 47 minutes. On a mixed diet, the test subjects pedaled 1 hour and 54 minutes.[5]

Legumes (beans, peas, lentils, etc.) are excellent plant food sources of protein. Protein can also be found in nuts, seeds, whole grains, and to a lesser extent in fruits and vegetables. Nuts and seeds include sunflower seeds, pumpkin seeds, cashews, walnuts, pecans, pistachios, macadamias, sesame (tahini), nut butters, peanuts, and almonds. Whole grains can include items such as brown rice, millet, barley, flours, pasta, granola, bulghur wheat, cereal, corn, oats, and couscous. Some examples of legumes (plants that house edible seeds within a pod that opens lengthwise) include navy beans, green peas, chick peas, soy beans, tofu (soy curd), lentils, mung beans, alfalfa sprouts, and kidney beans. Textured vegetable protein (TVP) and textured soy protein (TSP) are other sources of protein.

The concern that vegetables do not contain "complete proteins" is not scientifically valid. Plenty of protein and all of the essential and nonessential amino acids are present in single unrefined starches, such as oatmeal (16% of calories from protein), rice (8% protein), corn (12% protein), beans (26% protein), whole wheat spaghetti (14% protein), and potatoes (11% protein), enough even for weight lifters and endurance athletes, but very rarely exceeding the target for ideal health, which is only 15% of total calories from protein.[6]

On a high-protein diet, the liver and kidneys become burdened. Eventually, they enlarge and begin to take calcium

from the bones in an effort to alkalinize the acidity caused by
the presence of excess protein, and by the sulfur-containing
amino acids found in animal products. The amount of calcium lost daily exceeds the amount of calcium absorbed from
the intestines, resulting in a net loss to the bones daily. As will
be discussed in detail later, osteoporosis is often due to loss
of calcium from the bones, *not* lack of calcium in the diet, as
evidenced by reputable research done all over the world.

Compare the protein content of the starches listed above
with that of beef (26% protein), pork (42% protein), lobster
(88% protein), skinned chicken (61% protein), skinned
turkey (68% protein), and whole cow milk (21% protein). It
is also worth noting that sulfur-containing amino acids, like
the ones used to make the proteins found in animal flesh,
cause more calcium loss in our bones than do the proteins in
plant foods. For example, although kidney beans and cow
flesh both contain 26% calories from protein, the kidney
beans will be much easier on the human body.

• AMINO ACIDS

There are twenty-two amino acids that have been identified
as necessary for the health of the human body. The eight
essential (i.e., acquired through our diet) and fourteen
nonessential (i.e., synthesized by our bodies) amino acids are
all found in sufficient amounts in a variety of plant foods.
Plants, not animals, are the original sources of amino acids,
although many people believe that one must eat animals in
order to get amino acids. This is dangerous because of the
high protein content of animal flesh and products, as
described above.

• CALCIUM

Research has proven that the bioavailability of cow-milk calcium is inferior to that found in kale and other greens.[7] Cup for cup, calcium-fortified soy milk, calcium-fortified orange juice, and many leafy greens have about the same amount of calcium as cow milk (about 200–300 mg per 8 ounces), with an added advantage: vegan calcium sources do not contain cholesterol or saturated fat, or the animal protein that can burden the kidneys as they try to excrete it (see Protein, above, and Chapter 6).

Cows get their calcium from plants, and so can we. Excellent calcium sources include green leafy vegetables (except spinach and Swiss chard, which contain oxalates that inhibit calcium absorption), seeds, nuts, oranges, kidney beans, lima beans, whole grains, raisins, collard greens, lentils, garbanzo beans and hummus, cashews, almonds, tofu, broccoli, kale, mustard greens, carrots, celery, apricots, and romaine lettuce. One tablespoon of blackstrap molasses provides 187 mg of calcium.[8] Calcium-fortified tofu, orange juice, soy milks, rice milks, and other prepared foods are also available. Interestingly, Reed Mangels, Ph.D., R.D., found in *Vegetarian Journal* that most of the plant-derived milks he studied contained more bioavailable calcium than cow milk.[9]

• IRON

If the stores of iron are sufficient in the body, only about 5% of dietary intake (or 1–2 mg/day) is absorbed, compared to 20% absorption (up to 6 mg/day) if the body is deficient. Absorption depends upon the acidity of the stomach, the amount of fiber present, the presence of vitamin C, the kinds of amino acids present, the absence of caffeine and tannic acids, and whether the iron form is heme (also known as "organic," occurring in hemoglobin or myoglobin molecules in animal sources) or nonheme (also known as "inorganic," occurring in plant and animal sources). Many dietitians not yet educated in plant-based nutrition say that iron must come from animal sources in order to be useful to humans, but this is untrue. Vitamin C, which is abundant in many plant foods and deficient in animal foods, enhances the absorbability of plant iron, enabling humans to obtain adequate iron through a well-planned vegan diet.

Since about 1 in 20 menstruating women, both vegetarian and non-vegetarian, suffer from iron-deficiency anemia, regular checking of iron levels is prudent in this population, regardless of diet. Any decision to supplement with iron should be made with the advice of a physician. The potential for iron loss through menstruation is exacerbated by the fact that women on the typical, high-fat SAD have abnormally high levels of estrogens in their bodies, causing a thicker buildup of endometrial tissues in the uterus. At the end of each monthly cycle, when these tissues are shed, the bleeding from this overgrown endometrial lining is heavier and longer than it would have been at normal estrogen levels, resulting in a potentially greater iron loss.

In men, the most common cause of iron-deficiency anemia is through ulcers, hemorrhoids, and other abnormalities of the gastrointestinal tract.[10] The prevention and treatment of gastrointestinal injuries requires a switch from stress-promoting to health-promoting lifestyle factors, including a diet that is as free as possible of the harmful fats, synthetic chemicals, and food allergens that characterize the SAD.

Another consideration for followers of the SAD, or for lacto- and lacto-ovo-vegetarians, is that cow milk and its products have been shown to actually inhibit absorption of iron in the human body![11] Finally, it should be noted that iron-deficiency anemia is no more likely to occur in vegetarian than nonvegetarian children.[12]

Iron sources include legumes (beans, peas, lentils), leafy green vegetables (except spinach, Swiss chard, and beet greens), dried fruits, molasses, many whole grains, and iron-fortified cereals and grains. Many people believe that sea vegetables, such as kombu, hijiki, wakame, and nori, are also a good source of iron; however, the high iodine content of many seaweeds limits the bioavailability of their iron.

• FOLIC ACID

Because of the nature of the vegan diet, most vegans exceed the daily requirements for folic acid published by the government. Excellent sources of folic acid include dark green, leafy vegetables (like kale, collards, spinach, and romaine lettuce), Red Star Vegetarian Support Formula Nutritional Yeast, dates, broccoli, peas, Brussels sprouts, soybeans, navy beans, garbanzo beans, many cereals, orange juice, lentils, pinto beans, and asparagus.

• VITAMIN B12 (cyanocobalamin or cobalamin)

Vitamin B12 is made by bacteria and can be found in tiny amounts in our saliva, in the liver's bile, and in the intestines,[13] but nutrition experts caution not to rely on these sources, or on the often-quoted statement that our liver stores B12 for three to five years, to meet our B12 needs. Animals typically accumulate B12 in their flesh or milk by consuming manure, commercial feed, water, and B12-rich soil. However, the use of synthetic herbicides, pesticides, and other chemicals that have a sterilizing effect on soil and plants has all but eliminated natural, plant-based foods as a reliable source of this bacteria-driven nutrient, and the similar effects of pasteurization, irradiation, and other processing methods suggest that even those who eat animal flesh or drink animal milk should ensure adequate B12 from fortified foods or supplements. Many of today's prepared vegan foods and veggie, soy, rice, or almond milks are fortified with B12, as are other soy products, cereals, and Red Star Vegetarian Support Formula Nutritional Yeast, making this important issue easier to address.

Apart from dietary intake, impaired absorption may also be a risk factor for B12 deficiency. According to Brenda Davis, R.D., over 95% of cases of B12 deficiency do not occur in vegans and are not due to inadequate B12 intake. The inability to absorb the protein-bound form of B12 found in animal foods occurs in 10–30% of people over age 50, due to reduced gastric acid and pepsin enzyme secretions.[14] This is one of the reasons that Israel began a widespread B12 fortification program for bread and other wheat products in 2002.

Research shows that we require about 3 micrograms of vitamin B12 per day. The latest recommendation, according to Jack Norris, R.D., an expert on B12 and vegan nutrition, is 2,000 mcg sublingually once per week, or 10–100 mcg per day. Alternatively, an adult can eat two servings of B12-fortified foods, (at least six hours apart, containing at least 20% of the recommended daily value) each day. The Institute of Medicine recommends that infants of vegan mothers be supplemented with B12 from birth because their stores at birth and their mother's milk supply may be low.[15]

Dr. Michael Greger, an expert in vegan nutritional medicine, recommends the Urine MMA laboratory test (if high, then interpret B12 as low) as superior in accuracy to the more common serum B12 tests.

• VITAMIN D

Vitamin D is a main prerequisite to the absorption of calcium and phosphorus from the intestines and is therefore important in the remineralization of bones. It also helps to regulate blood clotting, optimizes the function of the nerves and muscles, and affects our skin, pancreas, glandular function, and immune system. Deficiency can result in diseases such as osteomalacia or rickets.

The groups of compounds that are important for humans include provitamin D2 (ergosterol and ergocalciferols), which is found in small quantities in yeast and in chanterelle and shiitake mushrooms, and vitamin D3 (precalciferol, 7-dehydrocholesterol, cholecalciferols), the form found in animals, fish, and humans. Unfortunately, the fats and oils that contain vitamin D3 often store several concentrated harmful environmental toxins.

Vitamin D is more like a hormone than a vitamin, as the skin synthesizes it when exposed to sunlight, after which it travels to the kidney, intestines, and bones to take effect. For non-elderly, light-skinned individuals in sunny climates like

Los Angeles or Atlanta and farther south, the general recommendation is fifteen minutes of mid-morning or afternoon sunlight per day on the face or forearms. Darker skin requires three to six times more sunlight than lighter skin to produce the same amount of vitamin D (with the darkest skin requiring the longest exposure), because in a given period less sunlight reaches the deeper layers of darker skin.[16]

For people who do not get sufficient sunlight, live in climates with less sunlight (i.e., north of Los Angeles or Atlanta), wear sunscreen, or are elderly (with a reduced capacity to synthesize vitamin D), Dr. Michael Greger recommends ensuring vitamin D intake through fortified foods or supplements. The current Daily Value (DV) for vitamin D is 10 mcg per day, with an accepted range of about 5–15 mcg (or 200–400 IU) per day.

Vegan food sources of vitamin D include shiitake and chanterelle mushrooms, fortified rice milk or soy milk, fortified cereals, and quality vegan multivitamin supplements. It should be noted that the vitamin D found in cow milk is added at the dairy plant; it is not present in natural cows' milk.[17]

There are great advantages to obtaining these nutrients first-hand from fresh plant foods when possible, rather than pre-digested and stored, along with huge amounts of contaminants, in the flesh of cows and other animals.

A brief description of a few other nutrients may also be helpful here.

• FATS

The word "fat" usually refers to saturated fats, which are solid at room temperature. Oils are unsaturated vegetable fats, which are usually liquid at room temperature. The only fats we do not have the ability to synthesize on our own are the essential fatty acids, which we can obtain through a healthy, plant-based diet.

• **CARBOHYDRATES**

The bad press attributed to carbohydrates in general, usually by high-protein-diet promoters, should really be confined to *refined* carbohydrates, which contribute to many of the chronic diseases discussed in this book. We see refined carbohydrates in packaged foods, baked goods, candy, pop, fast foods, and many flours, pretzels, crackers, and breads. Consuming refined carbohydrates causes a rapid increase in blood sugar, resulting in an immediate pancreatic insulin "spike" to bring the blood sugar back down, and usually contributes to excess fat storage.

Unrefined carbohydrates, on the other hand, are the human body's most efficient source of energy, and are necessary in the building of structural and functional materials. The body responds quite differently to balanced, whole foods than to refined carbohydrates. In whole grains, fruits, legumes, and vegetables, the sugar is combined with fiber. The fiber serves as a "time-release" mechanism, which helps to avoid drastic ups and downs in blood sugar. Eating these foods helps the body to correctly balance insulin and thereby to usher only the necessary amounts of sugar into the muscles, brain, organs, and other cells. Fruits, vegetables, beans, and grains with their fiber or bran intact, or whole-grain breads and pastas, do not cause a harmful sugar spike in the blood, but produce a slow and steady rise in blood sugar for constant energy throughout the day.

• **CHOLESTEROL**

Humans have no need for dietary cholesterol. Our bodies make sufficient cholesterol (600–800 mg per day) for the synthesis of vitamin D through the skin, bile acids through the liver, and hormones like estrogens, androgens, and adrenal steroids.

Dietary cholesterol is only found in animal products, like pork, eggs, beef, turkey, chicken, lobster, fish, cheese, cow milk, and buffalo. Cholesterol is not present in vegetables, fruits, legumes, or grains. Further, with the exception of a few highly saturated plant fats (cocoa butter, shortening, margarine, and coconut or palm kernel oil), all plant foods help to lower cholesterol levels in the body. Finally, natural fiber, which has a protective effect against hypercholesterolemia, is only found in plant foods, and never in animal flesh or fluids.

The United States Surgeon General stated in 1988 that the "highest priority" among dietary changes should be to reduce the intake of foods high in fat, and to increase the intake of foods high in complex carbohydrates and fiber. He highlighted the continuously graded positive correlation between high blood cholesterol and coronary heart disease, and referred to the many cancers that are sensitive to dietary fats. (Certain cancers grow faster in response to the hormone load stored in fatty foods, or when a high-fat diet inhibits the function of antioxidants in the body.)[18] But there are serious hazards in trying to follow the Surgeon General's recommendations in the context of the SAD.

First, when the saturated animal fat content is lowered in an animal-based diet, simple math tells us that the animal protein content will be raised. Every food item consists of fat, protein, and carbohydrate, the total of which must be 100%. Therefore, when the percentage of one entity is lowered, the other entities are adjusted accordingly, so that the total remains 100%.

Research shows us that excess proteins (especially animal proteins) are detrimental to human health in several ways. The current RDA for protein for human adults (0.9 g per kg of body weight) is easily gained from starch and vegetable sources.

In addition, people generally try to adapt the SAD to their "low calorie," "low fat," or "low cholesterol" needs by eating processed foods made with fat substitutes like Olestra, or artificial sweeteners such as saccharin and aspartame. While they attempt to cater to dietary requirements prescribed to treat such conditions as high cholesterol and obesity, these foods can contribute to other health problems, and they do nothing to foster an overall switch to a more healthful, plant-based diet. For example, a high potassium-to-sodium intake ratio is associated with lower blood pressure, and the ideal potassium-to-sodium ratio found in natural foods is 4 to 1. Processed foods completely reverse this ratio—1 to 4—a perfect set-up for hypertension.

Compared with natural foods, processed foods are strikingly deficient in nutrients. Compare whole wheat flour with "enriched white flour." Whole wheat flour (which retains its germ) provides 96% more vitamin E, 78% more fiber, 78% more magnesium, 58% more copper, 37% more folacin, 82% more vitamin B6, 72% more chromium, 52% more zinc, and 80% more selenium (note that selenium varies with geographical soil content). What is more, it has been proven that fiber, folacin, selenium, and vitamin E are essential nutrients that help prevent cancer.[19]

Most humans eating the SAD are also often depleted in fiber, phytonutrients (natural chemicals in plants that, we are learning, are necessary for good health but do not fit the definition of a vitamin or mineral) and other essential ingredients. All plant tissues contain fiber, but there is no fiber in animal flesh or animal products. Fiber is actually a long chain of simple sugars, which resists digestion because of its chemical configuration. Because it is not broken down in the digestive process, it gives bulk to waste products in the body, which helps the intestinal muscle (about 27 feet long in average adults) grab and pull waste through for efficient and timely elimination.

As stated above (see "Carbohydrates"), fiber is also necessary for the steady release of sugar and other nutrients into the bloodstream. This is one of the reasons that plant foods should be recommended for persons with blood sugar problems over the conventional medical recommendation of higher-protein foods like animal flesh. Choosing to eat animal products over plants also contributes to atherosclerosis, because fiber is needed to help "sweep" cholesterol, metabolic by-products, and other toxins out of the body. Excellent sources of fiber include Brussels sprouts, parsnips, blackberries, raspberries, dried dates, lentils, kiwi, flax, bulghur, wild rice, rhubarb, beans, cabbage, carrots, cauliflower, kale, radishes, peas, scallions, tomatoes, green beans, and whole grains like wheat, oats, barley, and corn.

Relying solely on synthetic vitamin supplements to make up for the dietary imbalances of SAD is a mistake. Simply adding a vitamin to the SAD, for example, will not counteract excessive intake of saturated fats and cholesterol. In addition, while supplements are helpful in those cases where a whole food source is not available or a nutrient must be provided at specified doses, e.g., as prescribed by a physician to treat a specific deficiency, whole food sources are superior to supplements. When we look at antioxidant capability (the ability of a nutrient to seek and destroy cancer-causing free radicals), we find research showing that the benefits of whole food nutrients are much stronger and more far-reaching than single supplements. For example, it only takes 60 mg of vitamin C complex from a whole food to silence as many free radicals as 900 mg of vitamin C in the form of a supplement.[20] Research has also shown that foods rich in beta-carotene seem to reduce the risk of lung cancer,[21] while high doses of beta carotene in supplement form may not.[22]

Recent evaluations of the vitamin E found in natural food and in supplements show similar results. It was concluded that 10 I.U. (international units) of vitamin E from food could silence as many free radicals as 800 I.U. of vitamin E in supplement form.[23] Natural food sources of vitamin E contain all four of its identified tocopherols or forms (d-alpha, beta, delta, and gamma), whereas most supplements contain only d-alpha tocopherol. Vitamin E adds resilience to the cell membrane, decreases mutation, and enhances the immune system. Just one whole vitamin E molecule can disarm up to 1,000 free radicals.[24]

It will be obvious to anyone who studies the mounting body of evidence in the literature that synthetic vitamins are simply no match for the vitamins found in whole, unprocessed, natural foods. The biological activity of synthetic vitamins and natural vitamins in the human body is not equivalent. Vitamins are organic, biologically active substances, made for the most part by plants and bacteria, which function like wheels within wheels, depending upon companion nutrients for bioavailability and use. For example, calcium relies upon other nutrients, such as magnesium and zinc, for its transport into human bone tissue. A whole food like broccoli contains all three of these nutrients, but many calcium supplements do not. While supplementation can be helpful when carefully planned with a competent physician or dietitian, a diet rich in plant foods helps us benefit from nature's principle that the whole is greater than the sum of its parts.

We see another example of this principle in our grocery stores. When we purchase an "enriched" grain product we are usually buying a food item that has been stripped of over thirty nutrients[25] during the bleaching and refining processes, and had an average of only four to eight synthetic nutrients added back in. With the germ (which carries its fatty acids) and bran stripped in this processing, you are left with only a tasteless skeleton of the original food.

Those vitamins that are not stored in the body and must be eaten daily for good health (i.e., the water-soluble vitamins, including B complex and C) can easily be found in a variety of green vegetables, nutritional yeast, and fruits. Fat-soluble vitamins (A, D, E, and K), which are stored in the liver, are found primarily in nuts, seeds, oils, leafy green vegetables, deep orange-colored fruits and vegetables, legumes, some seaweeds, and whole grains.[26] Experts generally recommend at least five to seven servings of these foods per week. For those who choose to utilize supplements, it would be best to take an organic, whole-food supplement, eaten with a like food to help increase its absorption.

Dr. John McDougall, a vegetarian and pioneer in the role of nutrition as disease prevention, states unequivocally, "A starch-based diet with the addition of fruits and vegetables as recommended in the McDougall Program is ideal nutrition for adults and children over the age of two years. All of your needs for protein, essential amino acids, essential fats, carbohydrates, minerals, and vitamins are supplied in optimal amounts for growth and maintenance. Requirements for vitamin B12 may be the only exception."[27] To this the author wishes to add a reminder of the importance of getting adequate vitamin D (see "Vitamin D" above).

As we examine the SAD, we see a diet that is high in fats, animal protein, refined carbohydrates, and cholesterol. It is deficient in fiber and many essential vitamins, minerals, and phytonutrients. The more we learn about the effects of food on health, the more clearly we see that the PCRM diet using the New Four Food Groups is the best diet for optimal human health, and for the prevention and treatment of the diseases covered in the following chapters.

1. Barnard, Neal, M.D., *Food for Life* (New York: Three Rivers Press, 1993), xv.

2. Physicians Committee for Responsible Medicine, *The New Four Food Groups* (Washington, D.C.: Physicians Committee for Responsible Medicine: April 1991), cited in Alex Jack, *Let Food Be Thy Medicine* (Becket, MA: One Peaceful World Press, 1991), 39.

3. Barnard, *Food for Life*, 147.

4. Fisher, I., "The influence of flesh eating on endurance," *Yale Medical Journal* 1907; 13: 205–221.

5. Astrand, Per-Olf, "Something Old and Something New . . . Very New," *Nutrition Today* 1968; 3(2): 9–11.

6. McDougall, John A., M.D., *The McDougall Program* (New York: Penguin Group, 1990) 43–45.

7. Heaney, R., Weaver, C., "Calcium absorption from kale," *American Journal of Clinical Nutrition*, 1990; 51: 656–657, cited in Jack, op. cit., 83.

8. Johnston, Patricia K., Dr.P.H., M.S., R.D., *Loma Linda University Vegetarian Nutrition & Health Newsletter—Ask the Experts*, Vol. 1, No. 1, 6.

9. Mangels, Reed, Ph.D., R.D., "Guide to Non-Dairy 'Milks' " cited in *Vegetarian Journal* magazine, January–February 1998, Vol. 17, No. 1, 19.

10. McDougall, *The McDougall Program*, 307–308.

11. Oski, Frank, M.D., *Don't Drink Your Milk!* (New York: Mollica Press, Ltd., 1983), 24–27.

12. Mangels, Reed, Ph.D., R.D., cited in *Vegetarian Journal* magazine, January–February 1998, Vol. 17, No. 1, 2.

13. Ellis, F. R., M.D., et al., "Veganism, clinical findings and investigations," *American Journal of Clinical Nutrition*, March 1976; 23(3): 249–255. Anonymous, "Contribution of the microflora of the small intestine to the Vitamin B-12 nutriture of man," *Nutrition Reviews* 1980, 38(8): 274.

14. Davis, Brenda, R.D., and Vesanto Melina, M.S., R.D., *Becoming Vegan* (Summertown, TN: Book Publishing Company, 2000), 135.

15. Norris, Jack, R.D., "Vitamin B12: Are You Getting It?" Revised May 2002, www.veganoutreach.org/health/b12rec.html.

16. Davis and Melina, op. cit., 135.

17. Klaper, Michael, M.D., *Pregnancy, Children, and the Vegan Diet* (Kapa'au, Hawaii: Gentle World, Inc., 1994), 13–22.

18. Koop, C. Everett, and the United States Department of Health and Human Services, Public Health Service, *The Surgeon General's Report on Nutrition and Health*, cited in McDougall, *The McDougall Program*, 170.

19. Pawlak, Laura, Ph.D., R.D., *A Perfect 10: Phyto "New-trients" against Cancers* (Emeryville, CA: Biomed General Corporation, 1998), 25, 87.
20. *The Berkeley Wellness Newsletter,* 1997, cited in Pawlak, op. cit., 120.
21. Shekelle, R. B., et al., "Dietary vitamin A and risk of cancer in the Western Electric Study," *Lancet* 1981; 2: 1185–1190.
22. *Journal of the National Cancer Institute,* 1996, cited in Pawlak, op. cit., 98.
23. *The Berkeley Wellness Newsletter,* 1997, cited in Pawlak, op. cit., 82.
24. Somer, E., *The Essential Guide to Vitamins and Minerals* (New York: Harper Collins: 1995), cited in Pawlak, op. cit., 98.
25. Jensen, Bernard, M.D., and Mark Anderson, *Empty Harvest: Understanding the Link between Our Food, Our Immunity, and Our Planet* (New York: Avery Publishing, 1990), 126.
26. Klaper, *Pregnancy, Children, and the Vegan Diet,* 19.
27. McDougall, John A., M.D., and Mary McDougall, *The New McDougall Cookbook* (New York: Penguin Group, 1993), 2.

3

OBESITY

THE CURRENT DEFINITION OF OBESITY IS GENER-
ally 20% over the ideal weight for men, 25% for women.
"Ideal body weight" has traditionally been defined by
Metropolitan Life Insurance data that find mortality rates of
insured clients lowest at these weights. Estimates vary on
obesity in America, but the National Institutes of Health
puts the figure at about 40 million adults. One third of the
population in all industrialized countries is considered obese,
and the United States alone openly attributes 300,000 deaths
per year directly to obesity.[1]

A 1997 report from the Colorado Health Sciences Center
shows that these statistics have been rising rapidly in our
country. For example, over 35% of adults are overweight
enough to be unhealthy—up from 25% in 1980. About 12%
of America's adolescents aged 12–17 years are overweight,
up from 6% in 1980. Finally, 14% of children aged 6–11
years are overweight, up from 8% in 1980.[2]

Sadly, about 95% of the victims of obesity go on diet
after diet, only to gain most or all of the weight back within
one year.[3] Americans spend over $30 billion each year on
commercial weight reduction programs and products,
including exercise machinery and fruitless gimmicks

designed for rapid weight loss—the proverbial "quick fix." Meanwhile, despite even the most drastic measures, from diets and herbal formulas to drugs and surgeries (such as intestinal bypass, gastric bypass, gastric stapling, and suction lipectomy), the success rate of conventional medicine in achieving permanent weight reduction is less than 10%.[4]

Obesity can negatively affect every aspect of human life, producing decreased mobility, emotional turmoil, low self-esteem, and feelings of intellectual defeat, not to mention organ failure, circulatory complications, stress fracture, stroke, heart trouble, and many other negative effects—including death. Recent reviews note health problems and increased mortality rates due even to mild cases of obesity.

Obesity is also statistically significantly correlated with several seemingly unrelated diseases.[5] For example, as weight goes up anywhere on the body, so does the incidence of breast cancer.[6] Some research studies have shown that obesity may be a major contributing factor in a nerve-conduction problem in the hand known commonly as carpal tunnel syndrome. (It is now being considered that occupational stressors may simply worsen, rather than cause, the problem.) Research from the University of Michigan on 1,300 adults found that people who on first measurement were 20% or more overweight were three times more likely to have osteoarthritis of the hands, when checked again twenty-three years later, than were slimmer people of the same age. The arthritis in the overweight group was also more severe.

Obesity alters one's overall quality of life, and it can affect the functioning of every system in the body. Complications related to obesity in the circulatory system can take the form of elevated blood pressure, varicose veins in the legs, strokes, erratic heartbeat, enlargement of the heart, cardiovascular disease, or heart attacks. Excess weight also intensifies snoring, sweating, and pains related to arthritis in the hip, knee, fingers, and ankle bones. Obesity has been linked to cancer of the gallbladder, cervix, breast, and ovaries. Diabetes, reproductive difficulties, kidney and gall stones, and cirrhosis of the liver have also been identified as complications of obesity.[7]

The results of a 12-year study in the *New England Journal of Medicine* add to the growing body of evidence that carrying extra weight (per Body Mass Index measurements) increases the risk of early death due to disease. The study of more than 260,000 men aged 30 to 74 years found that being overweight is particularly deadly for younger adults. After age 74, weight does not seem to influence the risk of death.[8] This last statistic may point to inherent genetic strengths in that subgroup of people, but it is clear to see that carrying extra weight in earlier years carries significant related disease risk.

Another example comes from doctors at the School of Medicine at Yokohama City University who researched immune function via blood tests in thirty-four obese people, pre and post dietary change. After an average weight loss of about 50 pounds, the T-lymphocytes (necessary in fighting disease such as cancer) nearly doubled in number.

Most theories regarding the etiology of obesity are rooted in the belief that thoughtless overeating is the root of obesity in all cases.[9] The author, however, proposes that if we accept the fact that every human body is unique in its combination of genetic strengths and frailties, which vary from culture to family to individual, we begin to see effective prevention, proper diagnosis and treatment for obesity as a responsibility for our entire society. For those not inclined toward social responsibility, the author points to the current costs to society of each individual's disability, resulting lack of motivation and energy for employment, loss of productivity, health care dollars spent, and years of governmental assistance.

Delineated below are the five viable etiologies to which this author attributes obesity in humans. Note that some etiologies are clearly endogenous (caused by internal factors), some are clearly exogenous (caused by external factors), and some are actually both.

1. Persons with a depressive state of brain chemistry seeking to elevate physiological mood via the stimulation of serotonin and endogenous endorphins through the act of ingesting sugars, refined carbohydrates, chocolate, caffeine, etc. This depressive state may be genetic or situational, or both.

2. Individuals whose brain chemistry is insensitive to leptin, the chemical that communicates that sufficient amounts of food have been ingested and sends signals to stop eating.

3. Individuals who have inherited a mechanism that tells the body to continue to store fat beyond the healthy and statistically normal range.

4. Persons who continue with poor family dietary habits, not knowing the full extent of the damage

those habits may cause. For example, "My mom smothered everything in butter, so I do, too."

5. Persons who consume calories (with special emphasis in the areas of fats, refined carbohydrates, and sugars) in excess of what would be within normal limits given their actual physical activity level needs.

While some of these etiologies suggest more of an element of personal choice than others, all five are explanations, not excuses, for obesity. An individual should take responsibility for his or her own health and do whatever is natural, necessary, and within the realm of common sense to avoid disease.

For many people, this means adopting a diet and exercise program in order to lose excess weight—but there are important considerations that must be taken into account if the effort is to be safe and successful.

Many argue that "very low-calorie" diets and high-protein diets are both destined to fail because much of the weight lost is often muscle and water. When not fed healthfully, the body may perceive that the poor nutrient density is due to a famine or deprivation state. The loss of muscle decreases the body's natural ability to burn calories, and the perception of deprivation slows down the body's physiological metabolic rate. Now the body steps up its storage of fat to ensure survival during the "famine" it senses.

In addition, diets high in animal protein (which are also high in fat, saturated fat, and cholesterol) may put the individual at a higher risk for kidney disease, osteoporosis, heart attack and stroke. Finally, any diet that touts a lifestyle that cannot be sustained for the long term is a setup for failure. For example, programs that require the exclusive purchase of specific commercial foods or severely limit the food items allowed (e.g., watermelon only, grapefruit only, cabbage soup only, etc.) are not sustainable lifestyles.

To avoid these pitfalls, we must understand that the human body functions best when unrefined carbohydrates are used as its main source of fuel. The PCRM New Four Food Groups, the Pritikin Plan, and the McDougall Program, for example, are based on unrefined carbohydrates for this reason. By weight, unrefined carbohydrates are lower in calories than fat. Further, a meal high in unrefined carbohydrates decreases one's appetite for the next meal, which the ingestion of fats does not do.[10]

What the ingestion of fats will do is cause fatigue, laziness, and sluggishness after meals. The ingested fats flow through the bloodstream, literally clumping together with blood cells and slowing the blood flow down. When this happens, these fatty compounds actually block some of the smaller blood vessels and deprive the brain and other organs of essential nutrients and oxygen. It takes the body several hours to dissolve the fats in the blood and either store or eliminate the cholesterol and triglycerides. However, a steady intake of fatty foods ensures that the body can never fully rid itself of the harmful fatty compounds and becomes stuck in a chronic disease "process."

A diet including about 10–15% calories from fat provides an ideal amount of fat for the body to store as fuel for necessary processes at a later date. Carbohydrates are the only other nutrients with storage potential; however, each molecule of carbohydrate must be converted into a molecule of fat before entering a fat cell. In contrast, dietary fat requires minimal work for placement into our fat cells. Eighty percent of the carbohydrate absorbed from the intestine is in the form of the simple sugar glucose, whose main role is to provide energy for immediate needs. Any unused glucose is taken to the liver, and a small amount is resynthesized into glycogen, which accumulates in all the major muscle bundles and is used for energy during exertion. Our bodies can store only limited amounts of glycogen, so most of the unused glucose is converted into fat and stored in fat cells called adipose tissue. While the number of fat cells in our bodies is determined by about two years of age, the size and shape of the fat cells changes based upon the amount and type of fat stored at any given time during a person's life.[11] And because our fat cells appear to be able to expand indefinitely on the SAD, our bodies do not seek to create ways to burn off excess fat calories from the diet.

As an illustration of the effect of dietary input and activity output on body fat mass (adipose tissue), envision a basic diagram of "input" (dietary fat and activity level) into a circle, which leads to a certain "output" (result). Utilizing this illustration, consider high activity levels and a low-fat diet as the optimal "input" for the "output" of a healthy body size and functioning level. Accomplishing only one of the desired "inputs" results in compromised "output." Conversely, note that excess dietary fat and little or no activity have the most detrimental effect—an "output" that results in unhealthy and undesired excess fat storage. If optimal input is about 10–15% of calories from fat, we can see how the government's generally recommended 30% calories from fat, which includes abundant animal fat, usually results in excess fat storage. Studies conclude that many patients actually get worse on the Food Pyramid–based diets prescribed for them by most physicians and dietitians.[12]

Note that disease risk is strongly associated with the amount *and* type of fat in the diet. If the primary sources of dietary fat are found in healthful whole plant foods such as avocados, olives, nuts, seeds, and soy, one can maintain excellent health even while getting up to about 30% of calories from fat. (Note that tofu, which is a processed food made from ground soybeans and filtered to a liquid that solidifies, is approximately 54% fat and is deficient in fiber.) As we have seen, nuts and seeds and monounsaturated fats such as olive oil actually have a protective effect within a healthy diet. However, when oils and fat are derived from hydrogenated and animal sources, even a lower fat intake (15–30% of calories) can result in an increased risk for disease. The following recommendations of the World Health Organization and the American College of Preventive Medicine help to clarify the need to maintain healthy fats and essential fatty acids, while significantly decreasing saturated fats and eliminating trans fats commonly found in the SAD. The PCRM dietary recommendations for overall fats are lower (closer to 15% of calories), inherently eliminating saturated animal fats and dietary cholesterol, and focusing on more healthful plant fats.

In March 2003, the World Health Organization released the recommendations for diet in the prevention of chronic diseases (Table 2).

TABLE 2.
WORLD HEALTH ORGANIZATION DIETARY RECOMMENDATIONS

Carbohydrate: 55–75% of energy
Protein: 10–15% of energy
Total fat: 15–30% of energy
  Saturated fatty acids: <10% of energy
  Polyunsaturated fatty acids: 6–10%
    Omega-6: 5–8%
    Omega-3: 1–2%
  Trans fatty acids: <1% of energy
  Monounsaturated fatty acids: calculated by difference

Reprinted from *Report of the Joint WHO/FAO Expert Consultation on Diet, Nutrition and the Prevention of Chronic Diseases* (Geneva, Switzerland: World Health Organization, 2002), 40 (advance final draft copy released March 3, 2003), by permission of the World Health Organization.

The American College of Preventive Medicine, another well-respected entity, issued the following statement in 2002: "[A] diet rich in complex carbohydrates from unrefined cereal grains, vegetables, and fruits; moderate in total fat and restricted in saturated and trans fat; and moderate in protein is advisable for weight control, diabetes prevention, and health promotion. The College specifically recommends a macronutrient distribution within the newly released IOM ranges, with approximately 55% of calories from carbohydrate, approximately 25% of calories from fat, and approximately 20% of calories from protein. Saturated and trans fat intake should be restricted, with the bulk of fat calories derived from monosaturated and polyunsaturated fat. The College further recommends a fiber intake of at least 24 grams per day, with additional benefit likely from levels up to 50 grams per day in adults with diabetes.

"The College notes that there is currently a lack of evidence for the claims of popular diet that unrestricted intake of all varieties of dietary fat, or of protein, is conducive to weight control . . . further, the College advises against such diets, and all diets advocating restricted intake of grains, vegetables, or fruits, as they are incompatible with the aggregate evidence linking dietary pattern to human health. Given the large population with, or at risk for, obesity, insulin resistance, and diabetes, dietary intake recommended for the control or prevention of these conditions must be consistent with recommendations for health promotion in the public at large. Fad diets generally emphasize short-term weight loss while neglecting considerations of long-term health, and are to be discouraged."[13]

In regard to healthy weight loss and management, note the comparisons in Table 3 of fat content for various dieting systems, compared to the 10–15% calories from fat recommended by many preventive medicine specialists.

It's easy for most diets that include animal flesh and milk products to double or triple that recommended 10–15%. Remember that beef (the "top round cut") at its lowest fat content still provides 30% calories from fat. However, the fat content of beef is usually much higher, as in "ground beef" at 60% calories from fat and "top loin" at 40% calories from fat. Further, adding just one tablespoon of cow-milk butter to a cup of mashed potatoes pushes the calorie content from

| TABLE 3. DIET PROGRAMS AND THEIR FAT CONTENTS ||
Program	Fat Content (% total calories)
Diet Center®	20%
Jenny Craig®	30%
Nutri-System®	27%
Weight Watchers®	23%

Reprinted from Barnard, Neal, M.D., *Food for Life* (New York: Three Rivers Press, 1993), 87, by permission of Neal Barnard, M.D.

140 to 250, and adding butter to popcorn elevates the percentage of calories from fat from 12% to 44%![14]

There are a few high-fat plant foods, like seeds (85% fat), nuts (80% fat) avocados (88% fat), coconuts (87% fat), and olives (96% fat). Nuts, seeds, and avocados are especially helpful when extra calories are needed (e.g., for pregnant women, children, and athletes).[15] There is also a growing body of evidence that nuts can significantly decrease cardiovascular disease mortality.

To the suffering souls who have experienced the "yo-yo" effects of fad weight loss, it is even more discouraging to find that these highs and lows are possibly more destructive than maintaining the obese weight that prompted them to begin dieting. Kelly D. Brownell, Ph.D., a Yale University psychologist and obesity expert, reported these results in a 32-year study on weight fluctuations and their consequences. Every time one loses fat, some lean muscle mass is also lost. Regained weight without exercise is only fat, therefore, the desired weight or healthy body composition becomes harder and harder to achieve with each cycle of dieting. Dr. Brownell's somewhat maverick summary based on her findings of health is that "people should not undertake a diet unless they are really ready not just to lose the weight but to keep it off indefinitely."[16]

A low-fat, plant-based diet can not only make it easier to lose weight and keep it off, but also has been able to re-establish balances in hormone and neurotransmitter levels that help correct depression-induced obesity. We now know that three important and abundant neurotransmitters (which transmit nerve impulses within the brain and can alter moods) have nutrient precursors (that is, nutrients that are essential to their biosynthesis): tryptophan to serotonin, lecithin and choline to acetylcholine, and tyrosine to dopamine. Studies have shown that protein-rich meals depress brain tryptophan, because tryptophan is carried from the bloodstream into the brain by the same transport system that carries other amino acids. These other amino acids are more plentiful than tryptophan in most proteins, so tryptophan "loses the battle" in attempting to cross into the brain. A high-carbohydrate meal, however, actually enhances the entry of tryptophan into the brain by releasing insulin, which lowers the blood level of the competing amino acids, allowing tryptophan to cross unimpeded into the brain.[17]

Tryptophan is so important because it is the nutrient precursor to serotonin. Normal amounts of serotonin help us achieve better sleep, increase our pain tolerance, produce a calming effect, and help regulate body temperature. Serotonin also helps to curb cravings for refined carbohydrates, or "empty calories." The American lifestyle—lack of fresh air and sunlight, improper sleep, tobacco use, and a diet high in fat, refined carbohydrates, sugar, and protein and low in healthful foods—is serotonin-depleting. This may account for many of the depressive symptoms seen in our culture. In addition, one of every three depressive patients are found to be deficient in the B vitamins, and vitamin C and selenium deficiencies have also been implicated.[18] A well-balanced plant-based diet with sufficient selenium contains plentiful amounts of these nutrients, without the harmful animal fat and protein. Low serotonin has also been implicated in premenstrual syndrome symptoms and in obsessive disorders. Foods that stimulate tryptophan and serotonin can trigger a feeling of satisfied appetite and contentment. For example, almonds, avocados, bananas, blue-red plums, dates, eggplant, kidney beans, lentils, papayas, passion fruits, pineapples, quinoa, tempeh, tofu, and tomatoes can help to stimulate the serotonin neurochemistry. By contrast, the consumption of stimulants like tobacco, caffeine, alcohol, and sugar can actually increase appetite, because these stimulate other brain chemicals like epinephrine, adrenaline, and norepinephrine.

In summary, switching to a healthful vegan diet can bring the fat from calories back in line with current recommendations, as well as providing useful calories—rather than the "empty calories" of "junk food" (which the body stores as fat) and the saturated fat and cholesterol of animal products—along with the nutrients that enable the body to derive the full benefit from them. Further, the phytonutrient content of such a diet has been able to correct the cause of some cases of depressive-induced obesity by re-establishing balances in hormone and neurotransmitter levels. The serotonin-enhancing lifestyle factors noted above are ideal partners in reaching the goal of permanent weight management.

1. Pawlak, Laura, Ph.D. *Weight Matters* (Emeryville, CA: Institute for Natural Resources/Biomed, 1998), 1.

2. Pawlak, Laura, Ph.D., R.D., *A Perfect 10: Phyto "New-trients" against Cancers* (Emeryville, CA: Biomed General Corporation, 1998), 17.

3. McDougall, John A., M.D., *The McDougall Program* (New York: Penguin Group, 1990), 379–380.

4. Yetiv, Jack, M.D., Ph.D. *Popular Nutritional Practices: A Scientific Appraisal* (Ohio: Popular Medicine Press, 1986), 256.

5. Bricklin, Mark, ed. *Your Perfect Weight* (Prevention: Rodale Press, Inc., 1995), xi–xii.

6. "Will eating less fat lower breast cancer risk after all?" *Tufts University Diet and Nutrition Letter*, 14: 2, 1996.

7. Bricklin, *Your Perfect Weight,* 10.

8. *The New England Journal of Medicine*, cited in *Veggie Life* magazine, July 1998, 12.

9. Pawlak, *Weight Matters*, 5.

10. Ibid., 131–132.

11. Simone, Charles B., M.D. *Cancer and Nutrition* (New York: Avery Publishing Group, Inc., 1992), 38.

12. Ornish, D., Brown, S. E., Scherwitz, L. W., et al., "Can lifestyle changes reverse coronary heart disease?" *Lancet,* 1990; 336: 129–133.
    Blankenhorn, D. H., Nessim, S. A., Johnson, R. L., Sanmarco, M. E., Azen, S. P., Cashen-Hemphill, L., "Beneficial effects of combined colestipol-niacin therapy on coronary atherosclerosis and coronary venous bypass grafts," *Journal of the American Medical Association* 1987; 257: 3233–3240.
    Brown, G. B., Albers, J. J., Fisher, L. D., et al., "Niacin or lovastatin combined with colestipol regresses coronary atherosclerosis and prevents clinical events in men with elevated apolipoprotein B," *New England Journal of Medicine,* 1990; 323: 1289–1298, cited in Barnard, Neal, M.D., *Food for Life* (New York: Three Rivers Press, 1993), 56.

13. Katz, David, et. al. "Diet in the Prevention and Control of Obesity, Insulin Resistance, and Type II Diabetes: American College of Preventive Medicine Position Statement." American College of Preventive Medicine, 2002.

14. Barnard, *Food for Life*, 99, 100, 102.

15. McDougall, *The McDougall Program*, 42–43.

16. Bricklin, *Your Perfect Weight*, 169.

17. Yetiv, *Popular Nutritional Practices*, 71–72.

18. Pawlak, Laura, Ph.D., R.D., lecture on *Alternative Medicine: An Objective View* (Emeryville, CA: Institute for Natural Resources, 1998), Troy, Michigan, June 1998.

4

DIABETES AND HYPOGLYCEMIA

THERE ARE AT LEAST 7 MILLION DIABETICS IN the United States, about one third of whom have not been diagnosed. The annual cost due to lost productivity and medical care is over $20 billion annually.[1] Ten percent of diabetics are currently dependent on insulin. Although genetic predisposition is important, environmental factors must be present in order to trigger diabetes.

The name *diabetes mellitus* comes from a Greek word meaning "siphon," with a seventeenth-century addition meaning "sweet," in reference to the primary method of diagnosis at the time—tasting the urine for sweetness.[2] Diabetes is a metabolic disorder in which the ability to utilize carbohydrates is lost as a result of a disturbance in the body's insulin activities. Insulin, a hormone secreted by the pancreas after food has been ingested, allows glucose (an energy source that our bodies derive from carbohydrates) to be utilized as energy or to be stored for later use. Insulin regulates blood sugar by working like a key that unlocks the door on each cell, so that glucose can gain access and provide energy to that cell. When this mechanism malfunctions, glucose accumulates above normal levels in the diabetic's bloodstream, and the kidneys' filtration of the bloodstream can become overwhelmed and fail. Additional urine is produced to help excrete the excess glucose, and the resulting copious and frequent urination leads to dehydration, an often insatiable thirst and/or hunger, weakness, and weight loss. These are all hallmark signs of the onset of diabetic symptomatology. Advanced disease victims also experience difficulty breathing and coma if left untreated.

Popular belief is that all diabetes is caused by abnormally low production of insulin by the pancreas, as seen in childhood-onset (Type 1) diabetes. The childhood-onset diabetic produces too little insulin or none at all, usually as a result of genetic abnormalities or injury to the pancreas by viruses, chemicals, or abnormal immune reactions. However, in about 85% of all early-diagnosed adult-onset (Type 2) diabetics, insulin levels have been found to be almost twice as high as in normal individuals. Type 2 diabetics produce plenty of insulin, but their ability to control blood sugar is somehow impaired. This impairment is most often related to poor diet, lack of exercise, and obesity. Indeed, 90% of all diabetics also meet the clinical criteria for obesity.

Prescribing insulin and diabetic symptom management pills for Type 2 diabetes can control the elevated sugar level, but these medications can also have side effects such as further weight gain or life-threatening hypoglycemia, while failing to address the underlying problem. Meanwhile, the disease continues to affect many of the body's metabolic systems; even with (conventional) treatment, diabetics go on to suffer from blindness, kidney failure, stroke, atherosclerosis, and heart attacks, according to many sources, including the final report of the University Group Diabetics Program. Other risks related to diabetes include high-risk pregnancy, limb amputation, and insulin shock (a state of acute hypoglycemia usually resulting from an overdose of insulin, characterized by sweating, trembling, dizziness, and convulsions or coma).

As this chapter will explain, the new approach to diabetes focuses more attention on fat intake than on sugar intake. The more fat there is in the diet, the harder time insulin has in getting sugar into the cell, and minimizing fat intake and reducing body fat helps insulin do its job much better.

The fundamental problem in diabetes is the body's inability to metabolize glucose fully and continually. This is a vital process in creating cell body energy. In diabetes, the cells of the body are starved of the glucose necessary for their function, because excess fats in the blood get in the way of the insulin's ability to bind with the cell receptors and "unlock" the cell "door," preventing the passage of glucose to the cell. When this sugar backs up in the system (a condition called hyperglycemia), it may cause labored breathing, vomiting, and dehydration. As the sugar goes unmetabolized, the body begins to call upon more fat stores for energy. Metabolism of the fat stores creates a by-product called ketone bodies— chemical compounds that when present in excess cause a condition known as diabetic acidosis. Diabetic acidosis can cause coma and death if not treated with insulin and the right kind of intravenous fluids.[3]

Another condition, known as hyperinsulinemia, can occur when the pancreas is prompted to over-produce insulin to help deal with the excess glucose now circulating in the body (or, in rare cases, due to a pancreatic tumor). This over-compensation may lead to hypoglycemia, or low blood sugar.

In other cases, even the excess insulin cannot effect the uptake of glucose into the cells. This condition has been identified as "insulin resistance," and common symptoms include headaches, fatigue, concentration difficulties, memory problems, dizziness, sweating, and mental confusion—symptoms that many hypoglycemics experience as well.

In insulin resistance, the high level of sugar in the blood from excess sweets and refined and processed foods is met with a proportionally high surge of insulin from the pancreas. This response is an effort to help the sugar gain entrance into cells, but the cells become unresponsive, or resistant. More and more insulin is produced, but the body cannot use it. Insulin resistance can be suspected in persons with a history of diabetes in first-degree relatives, obese patients (especially with abdominal obesity), and patients with a personal history of gestational diabetes, polycystic ovary syndrome, or impaired glucose tolerance.

As the pancreas continues to over-produce insulin, "Syndrome X" can result—a constellation of problems that includes elevated triglycerides, decreased HDL cholesterol ("good cholesterol") levels, high blood pressure, hormone imbalances, and cardiovascular symptoms. Typically, persons with Syndrome X lead sedentary lifestyles and tend to store excess abdominal fat. Dr. Gerald Reaven, a professor emeritus at Stanford University's School of Medicine, considered to be an expert on Syndrome X, states that there are two critical behavioral changes that can greatly modify insulin resistance. "The two most powerful things are weight and exercise. The heavier you are, and the more sedentary you are, the more insulin resistant you will be."[4] Left unchecked, the vicious cycle of hyperinsulinism leads to classically defined Type 2 diabetes and its associated risks, including heart disease and stroke.

Note that both juvenile and adult-onset diabetes are rare or nonexistent in populations with plant-based or starch-based diets. In the case of Type 2 (adult-onset) diabetes, this fact is easily understood, as the animal fats and oils that characterize the SAD inhibit the action of human insulin and lack the fiber that could bind to the sugars and allow safer excretion. Unrefined carbohydrates, in contrast, stimulate insulin activity and lower blood sugar. It is theorized that the childhood diabetes rates are better on starch-based diets because the burden of the fats and oils in the SAD are not present and cannot weaken the pancreatic cells to the point where a virus could win the battle.[5] It is also worth noting that mounting research indicates that cow-milk proteins stimulate the production of antibodies that destroy the insulin-producing beta cells in the pancreas. When 80–90% of the pancreatic insulin-producing beta cells are destroyed, Type 1 diabetes becomes evident. Several sources now link diabetes to the exposure of a human infant to cow-milk protein (bovine albumin peptide), which may trigger the autoimmune process and subsequent Type 1 diabetes. Researchers in Finland and Canada found high levels of bovine serum albumin in every one of the 142 diabetic children they studied.[6]

Dietary modification and treatment is fundamental to the successful treatment of diabetes, whether it be Type 1 or Type 2.[7] Our bodies are meant to produce sugar by metabolizing carbohydrates from healthy and balanced sources (i.e., whole foods), not by the ingestion of the refined carbohydrate sugars found in the SAD. On a starch-based, no-cholesterol, low-fat diet, childhood-onset diabetics usually decrease their insulin needs by 30%, their blood sugar levels become more stable, and their risk of other complications is significantly decreased. On this same diet, 75% of adult-onset diabetics no longer need insulin, and 95% of them stop needing the pills they take to manage their symptoms.[8] The diabetic patient and his/her doctor are referred to *The McDougall Program* (John McDougall, M.D.) and the Physicians Committee for Responsible Medicine in Washington, D.C. for further medical direction and information in this area.

The vegan diet can also aid in the treatment of certain complications of diabetes in some individuals. For example, diabetics are also at increased risk for developing gout, a disease caused by abnormally high levels of uric acid in the blood, caused by foods that are high in purines. Among the list of foods that are high in the offending purines, note the absence of vegetables, fruits, grains, and legumes: animal meat, meat extracts, organ meats, shellfish, anchovies, mackerel and other fish, roe, sardines, gravy, goose and other poultry, mincemeat, partridge, and baker's/brewer's yeast.[9]

Hypoglycemia, a blood sugar abnormality that sometimes accompanies diabetes, can also be treated by the vegan diet. Other than very rare forms of hypoglycemia associated with liver disease or stomach surgery, etc., the most common form is called reactive, or postprandial (after-meals) hypoglycemia. It is diagnosed by blood sugar levels lower than about 50–70 mg/dl, accompanied by symptom complaints. The traditional medical recommendation for patients with this condition is to eat a low-fiber, low-carbohydrate diet, high in animal protein. This diet does not solve the problem but in fact leads to further disease in the form of atherosclerosis, stroke, cardiovascular disease and hypertension.

The best way to control the hypoglycemic swing is to eat a diet high in complex carbohydrates and low in refined carbohydrates, with frequent small meals. While highly processed (refined) carbohydrates have a high glycemic index, low satiety index, low fiber content, and limited nutritional value, whole unrefined carbohydrates tend to have exactly the opposite characteristics. There is also evidence that high-fiber carbohydrate sources evoke modest insulin response, can help reduce postprandial glucose and insulin levels, and can attenuate glycemic responses to high-glycemic-index foods. Foods high in soluble fiber slow carbohydrate absorption and help to prevent swings in blood sugar levels. Research has shown that fruits with their fiber intact, although they contain a natural sugar called fructose, do not stimulate insulin secretion from pancreatic beta cells. If isolated sweeteners are used, foods and beverages containing fructose generally produce less insulin excretion than do glucose-containing carbohydrates. However, readers may note the recently increased media coverage of the consumption of high-fructose corn syrup resulting in fat storage and insulin resistance in sensitive individuals, and as a general rule, it's best to avoid processed sweeteners altogether. Another consideration is that sugar-rich diets are frequently deficient in the nutrients necessary to support healthy cellular function and insulin reception.

The vegan diet offers solutions to both of the recognized mechanisms at work in hypoglycemia. Plant fibers help regulate and stabilize the insulin-blood sugar problem. This is why it is important to eat as many whole plant foods as possible; processed foods with the fiber removed (such as applesauce) cause the pancreas to produce more insulin than whole foods (like apples) would do.[10] Secondly, the vegan diet is naturally low in fat.

In conclusion, the vegan New Four Food Groups is the best diet for Type 1 diabetics, because it helps reduce the need for insulin and other medications, and helps limit the damage to the internal organs. It is also the best diet for Type 2 diabetics, because it eliminates the offending excess fats and simple sugars of the SAD, and provides much-needed fiber. Finally, the vegan diet is best for hypoglycemics, because it eliminates the problems caused by the high-animal-protein, high-fat, low-complex-carbohydrate, and low-fiber SAD.

1. Barnard, Neal, M.D., *Food for Life* (New York: Three Rivers Press, 1993), 124.

2. Wagman, Richard, M.D., F.A.C.P., ed. *The New Complete Medical and Health Encyclopedia, Vol. 2* (Chicago: J. G. Ferguson Publishing Company, 1987), 509.

3. Ibid., 511..

4. "Dr. Gerald Reaven and Syndrome X," an interview by Robert Crayhon, M.S., cited at Designs for Health, Advanced Training in Clinical Nutrition, www.dfhi.com.

5. McDougall, John A., M.D., *The McDougall Program* (New York: Penguin Group, 1990), 335–337.

6. Barnard, *Food for Life*, 126–127.

7. Murray, Michael, N.D., and Joseph Pizzorno, N.D., *Encyclopedia of Natural Medicine—Revised 2nd Edition*, cited in *Energy Times* magazine, July–August 1998, 26, 61.

8. McDougall, *The McDougall Program*, 337.

9. Thrash, Agatha, M.D. *Eat for Strength: A Vegetarian Cookbook, Oil-Free* (Alabama: Thrash Publications, 1978), 44.

10. McDougall, *The McDougall Program*, 366–36.

5

ATHEROSCLEROSIS, STROKE, CARDIOVASCULAR DISEASE, AND HYPERTENSION

ATHEROSCLEROSIS, OR ARTERIAL PLAQUE DISEASE, is the leading cause of heart attack and stroke in the United States. It is also the main etiology of hypertension, and causes hearing loss, kidney failure, gangrene in the lower extremities, enlargement of the prostate, and impotence (note the current interest in Viagra among men eating the SAD). Therefore, when atherosclerosis is diagnosed, it indicates potential trouble with any of these related ailments.

Atherosclerosis affects the arteries in one of two ways. First, arterial plaques (made of fat, cholesterol, collagen, cellular debris, and possibly calcium deposits[1]) accumulate within the passageway in an artery, interfering with the normal flow of blood. The blockages eventually become so severe that the blood-deprived tissues that were once fed by that artery starve or die. Second, atherosclerosis causes degeneration of the artery wall, so that the walls lose their strength and elasticity. Eventually, weakened artery walls can rupture.

Atherosclerotic diseases of the blood vessels occur almost exclusively in parts of the world where the diet is loaded with fat and cholesterol, based on animal meats, dairy, eggs, and processed and refined foods.[2] Only about

5% of the population has a genetic predisposition toward heart disease, and a healthy diet is a good strategy in these cases, as well.[3]

Every day, 4,000 Americans suffer heart attacks.[4] Every year, nonfatal heart attacks total 1.25 million in the U.S., and more than 900,000 Americans die of heart disease. Almost half of these heart attack victims are women. Nearly one third of America's adults suffer from high blood pressure, which is a major risk factor for heart disease and stroke.[5]

A heart attack can take various forms. A *coronary occlusion* is a total closure of the coronary artery. This may be caused by fatty deposits that have accumulated to the point of a complete closure of the channel. A *coronary thrombosis* is a blood clot (thrombus) that has suddenly caught on the roughened, fat- and cholesterol-clogged artery walls. The blood clot closes off the vessel, and the death of the tissues that are normally fed by this artery cause a stroke or a heart attack. In about half of such cases, the victim dies. A *myocardial infarction* refers to the actual damage to or death of the heart muscle itself, resulting from an occlusion or thrombosis.[6] Angina, or chest pain, occurs when the heart is taxed by excitement or exercise.

While today's technology makes it substantially easier to diagnose and perform surgery on an existing problem, we are lacking in commitment to true prevention of these life-threatening complications. Dr. Caldwell Esselstyn, a leading cardiologist with the Cleveland Clinic Foundation, has termed the options typically offered to cardiovascular patients (coronary artery bypass grafts, atherectomy, angioplasty, and stenting) "palliative cardiology," or a "rear-guard, after-the-fact approach." Dr. Esselstyn suggests that patients also be presented with a plant-based diet as a potentially curative option, analogous to a "military offensive approach" to cardiovascular disease.[7] Atherosclerosis is caused by poor diet, poor stress management, lack of exercise, smoking, and heredity. Four of these five etiologies are controllable by the individual. Interestingly, the controllable risk factors of cardiovascular disease are the same as those of many other chronic disease processes; the change to a vegan diet and a sensible exercise routine can also help to prevent or reverse obesity, hypertension, Type 2 diabetes, hypercholesterolemia, and osteoporosis.

It should be noted that attempts to correct or prevent heart disease and the conditions associated with it through means other than dietary change have proven to be problematic. Simply staying on the SAD and swallowing a daily aspirin is not sufficient for prevention of disease. When thirty-one random trials using drugs (such as aspirin) to inhibit the action of platelets were conducted on 29,000 patients with histories of angina, transient ischemic attacks, stroke, and heart attack, an analysis found that such drugs can help reduce certain health risks in people who have a *history* of atherosclerotic problems, but that these same drugs showed risks (such as stomach bleeding and stomach lining irritation, anti-clotting effects that could lead to death, and increased risk of hemorrhagic stroke) that outweigh their use in someone who has not had a history of atherosclerosis.[8]

Common medical surgeries for heart disease, which include risky and costly procedures such as bypass (a detour around the diseased arteries supplying the heart), angioplasty (to push the partial blockages back against the artery walls), and endarterectomy (removal of the inside lining of a diseased artery), address the symptom but not the origin of the problem, which is thought to be the product of excess fat, cholesterol, or triglycerides in the blood, or (more likely) the interplay of these three conditions. Before discussing the role of diet in the development and treatment of these conditions, it may be helpful to explain them in more detail.

Hyperlipidemia is the presence of excess fat (lipids) in the blood. There are three kinds of fats: monounsaturated fats, polyunsaturated fats, and saturated fats. Saturated fat molecules are completely covered with hydrogen atoms; monounsaturated fats have room for one more pair of hydrogen atoms, and polyunsaturated fats have room for more than one pair. Animal fats vary in saturated content from about 30–50%. Almost all plant oils have a saturated fat content of less than 15%. However, a very few plant oils also contain a high amount of saturated fat, notably coconut (87%), palm kernel (82%), palm (49%), and cottonseed (26%).

When unsaturated fats are hydrogenated (i.e., heat and pressure are used to force hydrogen molecule saturation), up to half of the bonds in the hydrogenated fats become trans fatty acids, mimicking the molecular shape and action of saturated fats. Researchers recommend avoiding trans fats (found in animal fats and in hydrogenated and partially hydrogenated fats and oils) because of their stimulant effect on the liver to produce cholesterol; a growing number of preventive-medicine physicians advise using the largely monounsaturated oils like olive and canola, or water, herbs, or vegetable broths in food preparation. As reported by the

National Academy of Sciences, "There is a positive linear trend between trans fatty acid intake and total and LDL cholesterol concentration, and therefore increased risk of CHD [coronary heart disease], thus suggesting a Tolerable Upper Limit (UL) of zero."[9] A new ruling regarding mandatory listing of trans fat content within the Nutrition Facts panel was issued in 2003, and will take effect from January 2006.

Excess intake of polyunsaturated fat (found in safflower, soybean, sesame, cottonseed, and corn oil) has been linked to gallbladder disease, because this type of fat causes the liver to excrete more cholesterol with the bile into the gallbladder. This change in the consistency of the bile may account for the increase in gallbladder disease when people simply switch from animal fats to vegetable fats. Even higher rates of colon and other cancers may be attributed to the switch.[10] Excess dietary polyunsaturated fats are also implicated in cancer and immune system disorders, most likely because excess dietary fat tends to suppress our immune system.

Eating saturated fat, most always found in the SAD in the form of animal fat, has many deleterious effects on the human body in addition to its role in atherosclerotic disease. Animal fats clot the blood more than any other factor we contact daily, by increasing the production of prostaglandin hormones that cause the blood vessels to constrict (this may slow the flow of blood and increase the chances of clotting). The fat then enters the bloodstream, coats the blood cells, and causes the cells to clump.[11] Saturated fats also raise cholesterol, further clogging up the circulatory system. If these clots close an artery in the heart, a heart attack results; if the blocked artery is in the brain, the patient suffers a stroke.

Cholesterol, which is not a fat but a sterol, similar to wax, is associated with fat because, like fat, it is not easily soluble in blood plasma or water. It is found in human and animal cells, and it exists in equal proportions in both the "lean" and "fat" parts of animal flesh. However, peak concentrations are found in the organs and glands. It never exists in fruits, grains, vegetables, or legumes.

In an effort to illustrate the dietary cholesterol load on most Americans' plates, Table 4 shows the cholesterol content of various foods found in the SAD. It's clear that simply "switching to white meat" makes no difference in cholesterol content. Although the saturated fat content may vary in animal, bird, or fish flesh, the composition of flesh in general causes overall negative effects on human health. Some other

TABLE 4. CHOLESTEROL CONTENT OF SELECTED FOODS	
Food (3 1/2 ounce portion)	Cholesterol Content (mg.)
Beef	85
"Skinless white meat" chicken	85
Lamb	52
Mackerel	75
Pork	90
Smelt	89
Turkey	82
Veal	88
ALL plant foods	0

Reprinted from McDougall, John A., M.D., *The McDougall Program* (New York: Penguin Group, 1990), by permission of John A. McDougall, M.D.

high-cholesterol foods are chicken eggs, liver, lobster, shrimp, crab, haddock, and trout. An easy way to remember what foods contain cholesterol is to remember that cholesterol is found in muscle..

The current medically acceptable range for blood cholesterol levels in the United States is 150–200 mg/dl.[12] However, the average American on the SAD has a cholesterol reading of 210–220 mg/dl.

It is not only the blood cholesterol level but also the distribution among lipoproteins (a complex of protein and dietary fat) that affects the risk of disease. Elevated plasma triglyceride levels, for example, can be indicative of an excess of refined carbohydrates, sugars, and alcohol in the diet. (Triglycerides are basically fat molecules bundled in the liver, packed into Very Low Density Lipoprotein packages, and sent into the bloodstream for deposit into the thighs, hips, and abdominal area, for use by the body at a later time.) Hypercholesterolemia, or high serum cholesterol, may be due to a high level of Very Low Density Lipoproteins (VLDL), Low Density Lipoproteins (LDL, or "bad cholesterol"), High Density Lipoproteins (HDL, or "good cholesterol"), or any combination of the three. These various lipoproteins are syn thesized in different locations in the body, but mainly in the liver, and they have different functions. By far, the most common cause of hypercholesterolemia is an elevated LDL level.

LDL is actually cytotoxic (deadly to cells) when it is added to a preparation of smooth muscle and endothelial cells like those found in coronary arteries. But the addition of HDL to the preparation has been found to inhibit the LDL-induced cytotoxicity.[13] One way in which this works can be

seen in the liver, where it appears that LDL picks up cholesterol and carries it out to the periphery of the body, while
HDL does the opposite, bringing the cholesterol from the tissues back to the liver for disposal. Thus, HDL is typically
considered a beneficial "scavenger."[14]

It is generally agreed that, in addition to keeping serum
cholesterol levels low, we should be concerned with maintaining a proper ratio of LDL to HDL. Dr. John McDougall
warns that focusing only on the ratio, while ignoring the
total cholesterol, can lead many doctors and patients astray.
However, the best way to accomplish both goals is through
lifestyle change, including a change in diet. The effectiveness
of dietary change alone has at times been challenged; for
example, a study in the *Journal of the American Medical
Association* found that a diet containing 22% calories from
fat lowered LDL cholesterol no better than a diet of 28%
calories from fat.[15] This is because the reduction in dietary
intake of fat from 28% to 22% is simply not sufficient to
reduce chronic disease risk.

Therefore, be cautioned when the media report that a
"low-fat" diet does not reduce risks of chronic disease;
remember that they are defining "low-fat" too loosely to get
results. Remember, too, that a "low-fat" diet does necessarily include reduction or elimination of refined carbohydrate
intake, which causes a harmful rise in triglyceride levels.[16]

Another problem with manipulated and misunderstood
data is aptly represented in another study from the *Journal of
the American Medical Association*, cited by Dr. Dean Ornish.
This study concluded that fat-restricting diets can bring cholesterol levels down, based only on change in lipid counts.

They found (as did Ornish) that in people on vegetarian diets, HDL cholesterol levels go down along with the triglyceride and LDL levels. They concluded that this must be unhealthy; Dr. Ornish, however, states that maybe our current concept of cholesterol readings is too simplistic. All of his research patients actually improved on every measure of health, even with the decline of HDL.[17] It is the author's opinion that perhaps the body only manufactures HDL at levels at which it needs it. Therefore, as the body is cleansed and becomes healthier, it reads the signals for lower levels needed, and responds accordingly.

Each type of dietary fat has a unique effect on the overall lipid profile. Monosaturated fats tend to lower total cholesterol and LDL ("bad") cholesterol. Polyunsaturated fats tend to lower total cholesterol, HDL ("good") cholesterol, and LDL cholesterol. Saturated fats tend to elevate total cholesterol—both HDL and LDL. Trans fatty acids raise total cholesterol and LDL, and possibly lower HDL. The omega-3 fats tend to have an overall lowering effect on serum triglycerides.[18] Clearly, choosing monounsaturated fats and omega-3 fats, and avoiding saturated and trans fats, can help to deliver a desirable effect on most lipid profiles. This is what preventive medicine experts mean when they say that the amount and type of fat in your diet is important.

Table 5 features excerpted data from a report on boys aged seven to nine years by the 1991 National Center for Health Statistics, and shows a positive correlation between dietary intake of cholesterol and cholesterol levels in the blood (although other genetic and environmental factors may also contribute).

Country	Dietary Cholesterol (mg./1000 cal.)	Blood Cholesterol Count (mg./dl.)
TABLE 5. **COMPARING DIETARY CHOLESTEROL INTAKE TO BLOOD CHOLESTEROL COUNT**		
Ghana	48	128
Philippines	97	147
Italy	159	159
U.S.	151	167
Netherlands	142	174
Finland	157	190

Reprinted from Jack, Alex, *Let Food Be Thy Medicine* (Becket, MA: One Peaceful World Press, 1991), 105 by permission of Alex Jack.

Cholesterol level (mg. %)	Closure of 50% or greater of coronary arteries found (% angiograms)
TABLE 6. **CHOLESTEROL LEVEL AND RESULTANT ANGIOGRAM FINDINGS**	
less than 200	20
251–275	60
greater than 350	91

Reprinted from McDougall, John A., M.D., *McDougall's Medicine—A Challenging Second Opinion* (Clinton, NJ: New Win Publishing, Inc., 1985), 103 by permission of John A. McDougall, M.D.

Dr. John McDougall noted the following blood levels as indicative of specific problems: cholesterol that is 180 mg/dl or higher (circulatory problems), triglycerides near or above 200 mg/dl (heart disease and resistance to insulin activity), glucose levels near or above 120 mg/dl (diabetes), and uric acid levels near or above 7 mg/dl (gout, kidney stones).[19]

Table 6 illustrates the undeniable relationship between blood levels of cholesterol and closure of the coronary artery. The table shows the percentage of angiograms performed in three separate groups, which reveal closure of 50% or more of the coronary arteries.

The "average American" on the SAD with a cholesterol level of 210–220 mg/dl has a greater than 50% chance of heart attack and stroke, as well as a 1 in 10 chance of breast cancer if female, a 1 in 20 chance of colon cancer, and a 2 in 5 chance of gallbladder disease.

The effects of the SAD are being detected earlier and earlier. In a 1988 study, the average cholesterol reading for children in schools in Bogalusa, Louisiana, was found to be 300 mg/dl. These children ate a diet in which 38% of calories came from fat.[20] Even children as young as nine months of age can show the beginnings of atherosclerosis in the fatty streak deposits found along the walls of their large arteries. Every child who has been raised on the SAD, which offers cow milk, cheese, hot dogs, hamburgers, milk shakes, and French fries, has signs of the disease by the age of three,[21] and, according to Dr. John McDougall's studies, teenagers on the SAD show hard fibrous plaques (where soft deposits of fat in the arteries are joined by hard, fibrous scar tissue to form larger plaques within the artery wall). These hardened plaques are indicative of a serious chronic disease arterial process.

By young adulthood, the damage is extensive. A study done on 300 autopsied American male soldiers (with an average age of only twenty-two years) during the Korean War revealed that 77% of their hearts showed atherosclerotic disease in the coronary arteries. Thirty-five percent of the autopsy specimens showed hard fibrous plaques, and eight of the soldiers had nearly complete or complete blockages in at least one of the essential coronary arteries.[22]

A panel of experts under the National Institutes of Health concluded that "it has been established beyond a reasonable doubt that lowering definitely elevated cholesterol levels . . . will reduce the risk of heart attacks due to coronary heart disease."[23] Luckily, research has shown that when an individual switches to a starch-based diet, his or her cholesterol level will fall 30–100 mg/dl in most cases, within three weeks.[24]

The Framingham Heart Study, directed by Dr. William Castelli, cites a plethora of research that points directly to the reversibility of atherosclerosis by utilizing dietary change. One Framingham study involved 5,209 people for a period of forty years.[25] Other case studies in humans have been documented in which blockages in the blood vessels have been reversed over time if the cholesterol level in the blood is lowered. Castelli also cites a study of 18,000 vegetarians in California, which found that the subjects had only 15% of the heart attack rate reported in nonvegetarians, and 40% of the nonvegetarian cancer rate.[26]

Another study cited included the determination of ratios of total cholesterol to HDL levels. The recommendation after calculations is a target below 4.5 (4.5:1), which would effectively change the fact that heart attack is the number one killer in the United States. The accepted ideal ratio is 3.0; most Americans have a ratio of 4.6–5.7, Boston Marathon runners scored 3.4, and macrobiotic diet followers (mostly vegetarian) scored 2.5.[27] According to the Oxford Vegetarian Study of 6,000 subjects, lacto-ovo vegetarians scored 3.25, while vegans averaged a healthy 2.88.[28]

In a study funded by the Netherlands Heart Foundation, Dutch researchers compared groups of nonvegetarians, semi-lactovegetarians, lacto-vegetarians, and macrobiotic males. The results concluded that the most ideal cholesterol levels were found among the macrobiotic men and boys.[29] As we have seen in more recent data, the outcomes of subjects following a strict macrobiotic diet are typically similar to vegan outcomes. In a review of twenty-two studies from Europe, Australia and the United States that measured total cholesterol levels, performed between 1978 and 2002, registered dietitian Jack Norris found that on average, the vegan group scored 41 points lower than nonvegetarians, with an average of 160 mg/dl. The lacto-ovo vegetarians averaged 185.3 mg/dl, "fish eaters" averaged 196.2 mg/dl, and nonvegetarians averaged 201.5 mg/dl.

A Belgian study done at the Academic Hospital of Ghent University found similar results, and also noted that the macrobiotic men were healthy, not obese, had normal values of vitamins, minerals, and proteins, and had favorable hormone levels. They enthusiastically noted that this level of health was " . . . really fantastic, like children, whose blood vessels are still completely open and whole."[30]

Another study simply concluded that a low-fat vegetarian diet has been shown to reverse the atherosclerosis causing heart attacks.[31] Whether this is because of the vegan diet's elimination of the animal protein, cholesterol, and fats found in the SAD, or its addition of fiber, vitamins, minerals, and other phytochemicals, the message seems clear. (Phytochemicals can reduce cell proliferation and oxidative damage, lower blood pressure, increase the openness of blood vessels, neutralize free radicals, and reduce blood clot formation. While all plant foods contain phytochemicals, of which thousands have been identified, fruits and vegetables are our best sources. For an excellent overview of various phytochemicals and their benefits, the readers is referred to *Becoming Vegan*, by Brenda Davis, R.D., and Vesanto Melina, M.S., R.D.)

In one study, lecithin, niacin, Vitamin E, and Vitamin C were found to lower cholesterol, and to reduce the effects of saturated fat in the blood and arteries, when found in a diet of whole-food forms such as legumes, particularly soy.[32] In fact, the anti-cancer properties of soy were given research attention by the National Cancer Institute to the tune of almost $3,000,000, back in 1991.[33]

A study cited in the *New England Journal of Medicine* regarding the effects of dietary intake of soybeans on blood levels of cholesterol, triglycerides and low-density lipoproteins showed a decrease in all three readings. Eating 31–47 grams a day of soy offers 30–50 mg of isoflavones (a flavonoid found only in soy) and in this study produced a reduction in cholesterol by 9%, a triglyceride reduction of 10%, and an LDL reduction of 13%. Isoflavones have also been found to block estrogen receptors in breast and ovary tissues. Note that the average adult living in Japan eats 30–50 grams of soy protein daily.[34]

Dr. Dean Ornish's treatment studies have shown that atherosclerosis can be reversed without drugs and surgery, through a lifestyle change including a no-fat-added whole-food diet, exercise, group support, and stress management techniques. His diet plan is about 10% calories from fat, 70% carbohydrate, and 20% protein. The diet devised for the current prostate cancer study deletes all dairy products, due to their connection (via the animal protein casein) to cancer promotion. In another of Dr. Ornish's studies, angina and other chest pains dropped by 90% within a few weeks of starting the plant-based diet.[35] Unfortunately, the patients who were fed the American Heart Association diet and received traditional care, such as drugs and surgery, had an increase in blockages.[36] Ornish notes that an animal-based diet is high in oxidants and cholesterol, while a plant-based diet is cholesterol-free and high in natural antioxidants.

Medicare officials announced in September of 1997 that they would test the heart disease prevention program developed by Dr. Ornish on 1,000 patients nationwide. If after this test (now in progress) they deem the program effective, Medicare will consider reimbursement for enrollment. "For the first time," *Vegetarian Journal* reported, "Medicare has agreed to study in a demonstration project a nonsurgical, nonpharmacologic alternative approach to medical care."[37]

In 1985, Dr. Caldwell Esselstyn of the Cleveland Clinic began a similar study on twenty-four patients with disease in three vessels. Six of the original study participants were dis-

charged for noncompliance with the recommended no-cholesterol diet; this group suffered six new cardiovascular
events by 1998. At five years, 100% of the compliant
patients had full arrest of the disease progression, eight of the
participants had regression, and the mean total cholesterol
dropped from 237 mg/dl to 137 mg/dl. At the 12-year mark,
the mean total cholesterol was 147 mg/dl, and the compliant
participants had experienced *no* new cardiovascular events.
This is particularly remarkable because these patients had
experienced more than forty-nine cardiovascular events during the eight years preceding the study.

One very important tool in the prevention of heart attack
and stroke is the willingness to see hypertension for what it
is: a symptom of a diseased blood vessel system. Effective
treatment requires correction of the cause, not just the symptom. Over 80% of cases of high blood pressure are considered borderline to moderate, and can be brought under control through changes in diet and lifestyle. This form of treatment is far preferable to the use of drugs, as research has
shown that the side effects of drugs commonly used to
attempt to reduce hypertension are significant; in fact,
according to Dr. John McDougall, diuretics actually double
the risk of sudden death.[38] The Joint National Committee on
Detection, Evaluation, and Treatment of High Blood
Pressure has also recommended that non-drug therapies be
used in the treatment of borderline to mild hypertension.

High blood pressure affects about 15–20% of the adult
population in America and other modernized societies.
However, population studies of "traditional" societies such
as the Inuit, Polynesians, Bushmen, and Central American

Indians show no increase of hypertension with age, but note its correlation to the introduction of refined salt, canned meat and fish, sugar, and other processed foods. Such findings have led researchers to conclude that "clinical primary hypertension may be a preventable disease."[39]

Several mechanisms for lowering blood pressure with the aid of calcium have been proposed. Calcium dilates the blood vessels and lowers the resistance in the peripheral blood system, thus reducing blood pressure. While dairy products are continually touted as a good source of dietary calcium, they also contain saturated fat and cholesterol. Even "low-fat" or "skim" cow-milk products contain casein and whey, which have been implicated in osteoporosis, allergies, and other protein-related disorders. In addition, the author speculates that the combination of fat and the milk sugar lactose contributes to many blood sugar imbalances, as discussed in the chapter on diabetes. For many reasons, the consumption of dairy products is believed to be a leading cause not only of atherosclerosis, but also of complications like heart attack and stroke.[40] Note that the highest rate of death in the world from heart disease is found in Finland, and that the Finnish are also the most frequent consumers of dairy products in the world. Compared to Americans, the Finnish people have more than 1.5 times the mortality from heart disease—and consume 1.5 times as much dairy.[41]

Calcium tablets and other blood pressure pills only continue to mask the symptoms of the problem: too much fat and cholesterol in the diet. Until the *cause* of the disease is corrected, the danger will continue to lurk in the victim's arteries, no matter how long one manages to cover up or ignore the symptoms.

A word on salt, which has been implicated as a culprit in hypertension: current safe limit recommendations on table salt are about 2,000 mg/day, but most Americans average 5,000 mg/day.[42] However, simply lowering salt intake is not the answer to hypertension, in and of itself. In *McDougall's Medicine*, Dr. John McDougall cites four research studies showing that although some vegetarians include generous amounts of salt in their diets, tests show that their blood and urine sodium levels are not elevated.[43] It appears that salt alone is not necessarily enough to cause the hypertension, but is probably one of many factors that interplay in the SAD. However, excess salt is implicated in stomach cancer, osteoporosis, and edema (swelling), and it is especially hard on those with kidney, liver, and heart problems.

Vegetarians generally have lower blood pressure levels and a lower incidence of high blood pressure and other cardiovascular diseases than non-vegetarians.[44] Vegetarian diets are naturally high in vitamins, minerals, fiber, and many other phytonutrients still being discovered, which inherently provide the protection needed against these chronic circulatory diseases.

It is such a tragedy that although the medical field talks a great deal about limiting cholesterol, hospital dietary departments continue to serve high-fat, high-cholesterol meals to their patients and staff. It is not only unhealthy, but also a missed chance to show the rest of the community what a truly healthy diet looks and tastes like. It is also a lost opportunity to help get the fat out of our medical professionals' diets and waistlines so that they actually could look the part of health, motivation, and energy.

1. Pritikin, Nathan, and Patrick McGrady, *The Pritikin Program for Diet and Exercise* (New York: Grosset and Dunlap, Inc., 1979), 18–19.
2. Connor, W., "The key role of nutritional factors in the prevention of coronary artery disease," *Preventive Medicine*, 1972; 1: 49.
   Stamler, J., "Lifestyles, major risk factors, proof, and public policy," *Circulation* 1978; 58: 3.
   Editorial: "Diet and ischemic heart disease—agreement or not?," *Lancet* 1983; 2: 317.
3. Barnard, Neal, M.D., *Food for Life* (New York: Three Rivers Press, 1993), 48.
4. Ibid., xiv.
5. Bricklin, Mark, ed. *Your Perfect Weight* (Prevention: Rodale Press, Inc., 1995), 4.
6. Wagman, Richard, M.D., F.A.C.P., ed. *The New Complete Medical and Health Encyclopedia, Vol. 2* (Chicago: J. G. Ferguson Publishing Company, 1987), 430–431.
7. Esselstyn, Caldwell B., "Resolving the coronary artery disease epidemic through plant-based nutrition," *Preventive Cardiology*, 2001; 4: 171–177.
8. McDougall, John A., M.D., *The McDougall Program* (New York: Penguin Group, 1990), 348–349.
9. National Academy of Sciences, "Letter Report on Dietary Reference Intakes for Trans Fatty Acids," July 10, 2002.
10. McDougall, *The McDougall Program*, 318.
11. Ibid., 351.
12. Bricklin, *Your Perfect Weight*, 352.
13. Hesler, J. R., et al., "LDL-induced cytotoxicity and its inhibition by HDL in human vascular smooth muscle and endothelial cells in culture," *Atherosclerosis* 1979; 32: 213.
14. Yetiv, Jack, M.D., Ph.D. *Popular Nutritional Practices: A Scientific Appraisal* (Ohio: Popular Medicine Press, 1986), 105.
15. McDougall, John, M.D., citing the *Journal of the American Medical Association* (November 1997), in *Veggie Life* magazine, July 1998, 10.
16. Ibid.

17. Ornish, Dean, M.D., interviewed in "The Heart Healer" feature in *Veggie Life* magazine, July 1998, 28–32.

18. Pawlak, Laura, Ph.D., R.D., *Alternative Medicine: An Objective View*, 3rd ed. (Emeryville, CA: Institute for Natural Resources: 1998), 24.

19. McDougall, *The McDougall Program*, 65.

20. Berenson, G. S., et al., "Cardiovascular Risk Factors in Children and Early Prevention of Heart Disease," *Clinical Chemistry* 1988; 34: B115–122.

21. Holman, R., "The natural history of atherosclerosis. The early aortic lesions as seen in New Orleans in the middle of the 20th century," *American Journal of Pathology* 1958; 34: 209.

22. Enos, W., "Pathogenesis of coronary artery disease in American soldiers killed in Korea," *Journal of the American Medical Association* 1955; 158: 912.

23. N.I.H. Consensus Development Conference Statement: "Lowering blood cholesterol to prevent heart disease," *Journal of the American Medical Association* 1985; 253: 2080.

24. McDougall, *The McDougall Program*, 406–407.

25. Ibid., 318–319.

26. Castelli, William P., "Summary of Lessons from the Framingham Heart Study," Framingham, Massachusetts, September 1983, cited in Jack, Alex, *Let Food Be Thy Medicine* (Becket, MA: One Peaceful World Press, 1991), 46.

27. Ibid.

28. Appleby, P., Thorogood, M., Mann, J., and Key, T. "The Oxford Vegetarian Study: An Overview," *American Journal of Clinical Nutrition* 2002; 70(3): 525S–531S.

29. Knuiman, J. T., and West, C. E., "The concentration of cholesterol in serum and in various serum lipoproteins in macrobiotic, vegetarian, and non-vegetarian men and boys," *Atherosclerosis* 1983; 43: 71–82.

30. Vermuyten, Rik, *MacroMuse* (Fall/Metal 1984), 39, cited in Jack, *Let Food Be Thy Medicine*, 47–48.

31. McDougall, John, M.D., citing the *Lancet* 1990; 336: 129, in *Veggie Life* magazine, July 1998, 10.

32. Pitchford, Paul, *Healing with Whole Foods, Revised* (California: North Atlantic Books, 1993) 122.

33. Pawlak, Laura, Ph.D., R.D., *A Perfect 10: Phyto "New-trients" against Cancers* (Emeryville, CA: Biomed General Corporation, 1998) 67.

34. Pawlak, Laura, Ph.D., R.D., lecture on *Alternative Medicine: An Objective View* (Emeryville, CA: Institute for Natural Resources, 1998), Troy, Michigan, June 1998, citing research by J. W. Anderson in the *New England Journal of Medicine* 1995; 333: 276.

35. Ornish, Dean, M.D., interviewed by *Veggie Life* magazine, 28–32.

36. Ornish, Dean, M.D., et al., "Can Lifestyle Changes Reverse Coronary Heart Disease?," *Lancet* 1990; 336: 129–133.

37. Vogel, Michael, "Medicare to Test Ornish Program," cited in *Vegetarian Journal*, January–February 1998, Vol. 17, No. 1, 22.

38. McDougall, *The McDougall Program*, 363.

39. Page, Lot B., M.D., "Epidemiologic evidence on the etiology of human hypertension and its possible prevention," *American Heart Journal* 1976; 91: 527–534.

40. Viikari, J., "Multicenter study of atherosclerosis precursors in Finnish children—pilot study of 8-year old boys," *Annals of Clinical Research* 1982; 14: 103.

    Hartroft, W., "The incidence of coronary artery disease in patients treated with Sippy diet," *American Journal of Clinical Nutrition* 1964; 15: 205.

    Oski, F., "Is bovine milk a health hazard?" *Pediatrics* 1985; 75 (Supplement): 182.

41. Truswell, A., "ABC of Nutrition. Reducing the risk of coronary heart disease," *British Medical Journal* 1985; 291: 34.

    Food Balance Sheets, 1979–1981, Average, Rome: Food and Agriculture Organization of the United Nations, 1984.

42. McDougall, *The McDougall Program*, 47.

43. Burr, M., "Plasma cholesterol and blood pressure in vegetarians," *Journal of Human Nutrition* 1981; 35: 437.

    Armstrong, B., "Urinary sodium and blood pressure in vegetarians," *American Journal of Clinical Nutrition* 1979; 32: 2472.

    Ophir, O., "Low blood pressure in vegetarians: the possible role of potassium," *American Journal of Clinical Nutrition* 1983; 37: 755.

    Sacks, F. M., Rosner, B., and Kass, E. H., "Blood pressure in vegetarians," *American Journal of Epidemiology* 1974; 100: 390–398.

44. Murray, Michael, N.D., and Joseph Pizzorno, N.D., *Encyclopedia of Natural Medicine—Revised 2nd Edition*, cited in *Energy Times* magazine, July–August 1998 24–25.

    Sacks, et al., "Blood Pressure in Vegetarians," 390–398.

6

OSTEOPOROSIS

OSTEOPOROSIS IS A METABOLIC DISORDER marked by porousness and fragility of the bones. The weakened bones result in postural changes and in fractures that occur under very little stress, such as coughing or taking a step. About 15–20 million persons are affected by osteoporosis in this country alone, and the diagnosis and care of people suffering from this disease has become a $4 billion-a-year business in the United States.

Throughout our lives, bone material everywhere in the body is constantly being formed and broken down. Osteoporosis, however, progresses at a rate of degeneration of about 0.5–2% of the skeleton per year. This often results in significant bone loss by age 65, while other systems of the body may continue to function well to at least age 85.[1]

While conventional medicine continues to advertise (seemingly on behalf of the dairy industry), that osteoporosis is a condition caused by humans not ingesting enough calcium from cows' milk, the Physicians Committee for Responsible Medicine and other physicians highly educated in nutrition have proposed a very different etiology based on comparative dietary intake studies. They support the theory that the primary cause of osteoporosis, the loss of calcium from bones, is the body's need to buffer excessive intake of animal protein, and *not* a dietary lack of calcium. Many societies that observe traditional plant-based dietary practices suffer less from this disease.[2] A great deal of the literature attempting to show that added dietary calcium strengthens the bones, or even enters them, has been unsuccessful.[3] We now know that having and keeping strong bones is a more complex issue involving an interplay of factors, including adequate calcium and companion nutrient intake, exercise and absorbability, and minimizing the excretion of bone material into our urine by reducing excess sodium or animal protein intake. Research attempting to correlate dietary calcium intake to bone density has been inconsistent overall, and there are other factors—including cultural differences (e.g., customs in Asia dictate that the elderly do not go for walks alone), climatic differences (e.g., slippery surfaces in snowy, icy regions), and genetic differences (e.g., Asians may tend to have shorter hip bones that are therefore biomechanically more resistant to breakage)—to consider when looking at hip fracture rates. For example, while research has shown that the Bantu may metabolize calcium better, and have better bone density, than other ethnic groups, other factors must also play a role, as illustrated in the lower osteoporosis rate of Bantu women in Africa when compared to Bantu living in the U.S.

Dr. McDougall states, "A consistent conclusion published in the scientific literature is clear: *Calcium deficiency of dietary origin is unknown in humans.*" He believes that the high animal protein content of dairy products actually promotes the excretion of calcium from our bones in efforts to digest the proteins, especially as seen in the case of sodium-rich cheddar cheese. This may explain how the United States, Finland, England, Israel, and Sweden have both the highest intakes of cow-milk products *and* the highest rates of osteoporosis in the world. Traditional Asian and African societies, with the exception of East African nomadic groups like the Maasai, who do consume cows' milk, typically wean children from human breast milk without switching to the milk of another species, and consume very few animal proteins.[4] (Note that people of African descent now living in America, Europe, and the Caribbean came primarily from West Africa.)

Animal products are a problem not only because of their high overall protein content but also because animal flesh is high in sulfur-containing amino acids. As Dr. McDougall has stated, these sulfur-containing amino acids are metabolized toward sulfuric acid, which the human body does not tolerate well. In the presence of excess sulfur, our body calls upon the phosphorus in our skeleton to serve as a "buffer" or neutralizer for the acid. We lose calcium in the process because it is calcium phosphate that is called upon to neutralize the acid. The excretion of this calcium and phosphorus load in the urine may contribute to kidney stones and osteoporosis, while the consumption of plant foods does not have this negative calcium balance effect; plant foods do not contain sulfur amino acids. Some nutrition experts have noted the health benefits of a diet based upon acidity, eating "freely" of base-forming foods and "sparingly" of the acid-forming foods. The vast majority of the acid foods implicated were animal products such as seafood, eggs, beef, poultry, and lamb. The base foods were a list dominated heavily by vegetables and fruits.[5]

A Michigan State study concluded that by age 65, meateating women had lost one third of their skeletal structures. Vegetarian women had less than half the bone loss, were less likely to break bones, healed their bones more quickly, and maintained erect postures.[6] More recent studies show varying results. Strict experimental controls for related factors, such as intake of caffeine, salt, and processed and refined vegetarian food products (elements that can make an otherwise healthful, whole-food, animal-free diet into an unhealthful diet) are important in producing a true picture of the difference in bone health between vegetarians and meat eaters. In 1998, the National Osteoporosis Foundation stated that the following factors should be modified to reduce the risk of development of osteoporosis: cigarette smoking, physical inactivity, and intake of alcohol, caffeine, sodium, animal protein, and calcium. For optimal bone health, vegetarians and nonvegetarians alike need to ensure an adequate dietary intake of nutrient-dense calories, containing bone-building minerals like calcium, boron, magnesium, and vitamin D, and adequate (not excess) protein. Caffeine and alcohol intake, and consumption of sodium and animal foods, should be limited. Maintaining lower blood estrogen levels, as naturally occurs with a healthful vegan diet when switching from the SAD, is also helpful.

The *Journal of the American Dietetic Association* published an article in June 2003 stating that "[T]here may be an advantage to including more plant sources of calcium in diets because research suggests that other compounds in plant foods, such as isoflavones in soy foods and potassium and vitamin K in fruits and vegetables, may favorably impact bone health." The authors went on to add, "It should be noted that this approach of emphasizing the variety of calcium-rich foods in different food groups is not specific to the needs of vegetarians but could be adopted for those who consume nonvegetarian diets as well. The advantages of this approach are relevant for all consumers regardless of diet choices."[7]

Scientists studying the Inuit Eskimo in Alaska have concluded that their tremendously high osteoporosis rate is attributable to the acidic effects of their high-meat dietary intake.[8] While they consume 2,200 mg of calcium daily from fish bone, the Inuit Eskimo have the highest rates of osteoporosis of any population in the world. Perhaps this high incidence is related to their daily intake of 250–400 grams of protein from fish—a quantity far in excess of the average adult requirement of 60 grams per day. Even frozen Eskimo bodies from over 500 years ago show the symptoms of severe osteoporosis.[9] And the United States as a nation ranks #1 (tied with Scandinavian countries) in the incidence of osteoporosis when compared to the rest of the world's nations.[10]

The amount of calcium in bones is very carefully regulated by hormones, and increasing the dietary intake beyond adequate levels does not fool the hormones into building more bone. Further, efforts to combat osteoporosis by increasing the intake of dairy products is not ideal, because many people are either allergic to cow-milk protein or lactose-intolerant. When we consider yet other concerns, such as the transmission of viruses and other contaminants in milk (which will be further discussed below), it seems clear that cow milk is not required in a healthy human diet. Cow milk has also been implicated heavily in eczema, psoriasis, cancer, rheumatoid arthritis, and atherosclerosis.[11]

Note that humans are the only species on Earth that drinks the milk of another species, never truly "weaning" our bodies as we are constructed to do after infancy. Rather than weaning, many people on the SAD merely switch from human breast milk to cows' milk. It might have made a bit more sense for us to drink monkey or ape milk, since we are more closely genetically related to these animals, but whether the milk comes from a monkey or a cow, it is not necessary in our diet. Standard whole cow milk turns a 45- to 100-pound calf into a 300- to 600-pound cow in one year. It is slightly over 90% water, 3% butterfat, and 2% protein (mostly casein, a substance that can form hard curds in the stomach, unlike lactalbumin, the protein in human milk, which human infants digest easily). The bovine protein, butterfat, lactose sugar, and chemical contaminants in cows' milk have all been identified as substances that cause ill health in humans; in addition, bovine leukemia viruses can be found in 20% of American milking cows.[12]

Interestingly, the advertisers of Enfamil, a formula marketed for infants, state in their own brochure, "Cow's milk is not recommended for babies for several reasons: . . . too much protein . . . the protein and fat are hard for babies to digest . . . too much sodium . . . too little vitamin C, copper, and iron, and . . . it can form a hard curd in the baby's stomach, causing digestive problems." At the same time, however, it offers three formulas that are cow-milk–based and only one that is soy-based.[13] Physicians and dietitians now state unequivocally the inadequacy and dangers of cows' milk for human infants, the American Academy of Pediatrics recommends no cows' milk for infants under age one, and Dr. Benjamin Spock advocated soy milk over cows' milk. It would be reasonable to ask why, in light of these recommendations, soy milk formulas are not advocated more commonly than cow-milk formulas.

Many researchers and physicians point to bovine proteins as the leading cause of food allergies. The most common symptom of allergic reaction is excessive mucus production, as the body attempts to trap the invading foreign substances. After consuming a cow-milk ice-cream cone, people will automatically reach for a glass of water to wash out the mucus buildup in the throat, and many vegans can detect this mucus buildup when they have mistakenly ingested a food with a dairy ingredient. Recurrent visits to the doctor for bronchitis, ear infections, asthma, sore throat, hoarseness, runny nose and other allergy symptoms are attributed to the feeding of cow milk to infants and children. However, although much of this data has been around for decades, some physicians continue to "prescribe" cow-milk formulas and lots of dairy products to our youth and their parents[14]—all of this in the midst of knowing that cow milk, chicken egg, peanut, and soy account for almost 90% of the food allergies in the first few years of our children's lives.[15]

Further, cow milk has been shown to irritate the intestines of many infants and children to the point of inducing low-grade bleeding, which can contribute to anemia.[16] However, the majority of American physicians prescribe a cow-milk formula with added iron whenever symptoms of infant anemia appear, without tracing the etiology.

Much of the "colic" in babies is a direct result of cow-milk protein and lactose fed to the baby either directly or through the lactating mother's milk. One good way to prevent or cure colic may be to take the infant off of cows' milk products and to change the breastfeeding mother's diet.[17] A study at Washington University found that babies with colic had mothers with significantly higher levels of cow antibodies in their breast milk.[18]

Some researchers see the problem with cows' milk primarily from the standpoint of its lactose content. Lactose intolerance is a condition wherein lactose cannot be digested due to a lack of the enzyme lactase. It affects most human adults (90% of Asians, 90% of blacks, 20% of whites, 60% of Mexicans, 60% of Eskimos).[19] Lactose intolerance results in symptoms such as cramps, diarrhea (sometimes leading to dehydration), and bloating. Products sold to promote the digestion of lactose (i.e., lactase) unfortunately increase exposure to a prime dietary source of cholesterol, saturated fat, hormones, and potentially allergy-triggering proteins. In addition, a case-control study cited in the *Lancet* in 1989 stated that "World wide, ovarian cancer risk is strongly correlated with lactase persistence and per capita milk consumption."[20]

Lactose has even been associated with vision problems, such as cataracts. In the digestive tract, lactose breaks apart into galactose and glucose. When galactose blood concentrations increase, the galactose can pass into the lens of the eye, where it degrades into molecular waste products that can lead to opacities of the lens. Humans have some capacity to break down galactose as infants, but we are meant to be weaned, and hence to stop ingesting galactose, after infancy. Some infants born with a genetic defect in their ability to metabolize galactose form cataracts within their first year of life.[21]

In terms of overall health, many preventive medicine practitioners say the consumption of cow milk to treat or prevent osteoporosis is like taking one step forward and two steps backward with each swallow. Even if one's diet is lacking in calcium, the problem can be solved with a healthful plant-based diet, without resorting to animal products. Approximately 45% (40–60% in many greens) of the calcium in plant foods is absorbed by humans, while the calcium found in animal foods is absorbed at a rate of about 30%. In addition, calcium loss can occur for hours after the ingestion of a meal containing concentrated protein, like cow, lamb, poultry, and fish, as the kidneys lose calcium in cleansing the blood of excess protein waste.[22]

Excess dietary calcium can cause kidney stones, calcium deposits in arteries, and impaired absorption of iron, zinc, and magnesium. The calcium found in fruits, grains, and vegetables does not produce these problems. Evidence has shown that when the factors causing osteoporosis are corrected, the process of osteoporosis can be slowed or reversed. The bones actually begin to remineralize. Unfortunately, however, once severe damage is done, acquired deformities are not corrected.[23]

Contaminants found in cow milk are also of concern. As of this writing, bovine tuberculosis (such as that found in northern Michigan herds in early 1998), salmonellosis, campylobacteriosis, bovine spongiform encephalopathy ("mad cow disease"), bovine AIDS (BIV), and bovine leukemia viruses (BLV) have been identified as threats to human health. Although some contaminants (e.g., salmonella, tuberculosis bacteria, BLV, and BIV) are killed by pasteurization, others continue to be found in the cow milk sold on supermarket shelves. I believe the high incidence of contamination is basically due to the thoughtless injection and feeding of cocktails of hormones, antibiotics, pesticides, and herbicides, which disrupt nature's inherent balances. (For further discussion of these contaminants, see Chapter 8.) In contrast, the vast majority of bacteria (one-celled microscopic organisms), fungi, and viruses that infect plant hosts are so different from those that infest animal hosts that they do not harm humans.[24]

Frighteningly, there is a growing body of evidence that many human leukemia cases could be linked to bovine leukemia. Bethwaite, et al., cites research from throughout the 1980s and '90s in American, Scandinavian, and New Zealand journals documenting the transmission of leukemia from cows to humans, especially in workers in the cattle industry. The highest rate of leukemia found, based upon occupation, is in dairy farmers, and also in the sub-population of children aged three to thirteen—the most frequent consumers of dairy products in our country.[25] This news is especially tragic when seen in light of the fact that humans absolutely have no nutritional requirement for cows' milk.

Finally, the prescription of estrogen to treat osteoporosis needs to be addressed. As of October, 2002, about 8 million women were on hormone therapy prescriptions.[26] However, estrogen therapy is not the answer to the osteoporosis epidemic. Taking estrogen supplements will slow bone loss but will not cause bone tissue to regenerate. In addition, estrogen therapy has been shown to increase the risk of cancer of the uterus by five to fourteen times, the risk of breast cancer by two times, and the risk of gallbladder disease by four times.[27] In 2002, the National Institutes of Health released facts about a study that was ended abruptly after 5.2 years, which tested an estrogen-progestin combination thought to reduce the risk of bone fractures. While it did in fact reduce the risk of fractures and colorectal cancer, it actually increased heart attacks, stroke, blood clots, and breast cancer. A safer approach in seeking answers to hormone questions would be to look instead at lifestyle factors that interrupt healthy functioning and survival, and to learn from other cultures. For example, women on the traditional plant-based diet in Japan have the lowest incidence of hot flashes in the world.[28] Many speculate that this is due to their high intake of fiber, phytoestrogen, or isoflavone, and their low intake of dairy products.

Exercise and use of the bones is the other key element to avoiding osteoporosis, as evidenced by studies on astronauts at NASA, pre- and post-flight. In an atmosphere devoid of gravitational pull, the bones have no weight to bear, and therefore actually begin to dissolve. Anyone who has had a broken bone casted has experienced some shrinkage of bone mass (and muscle mass) from underuse during the healing time spent immobile in a cast.

Combined with adequate exercise, then, switching to the vegan New Four Food Groups, which provide plenty of high-quality calcium (appropriate sources of calcium are listed in Chapter 2), and none of the offending animal proteins or animal amino acids, is the best strategy for osteoporosis prevention and treatment.

1. McDougall, John A., M.D., *McDougall's Medicine—A Challenging Second Opinion* (Clinton, New Jersey: New Win Publishing, Inc., 1985), 63.

2. Ibid., 62.
   Solomon, L. "Osteoporosis and fracture of the femoral neck in the South African Bantu," *Journal of Bone Joint Surgery* 1968; 50B: 2.

3. Kanis, J., "Calcium supplementation of the diet—I and II. Not justified by present evidence." *British Medical Journal* 1989; 298: 137, 205, cited in McDougall, John A., M.D., *The McDougall Program* (New York: Penguin Group, 1990), 383 .
   Heaney, R. "Calcium nutrition and bone health in the elderly American," *Journal of Clinical Nutrition* 1982; 36: 986.
   Draper, H., "Calcium, phosphorous, and osteoporosis," *Fed. Proc.* 1981; 40: 2434 .

4. McDougall, *The McDougall Program*, 48.

5. Thrash, Agatha, M.D. *Eat For Strength: A Vegetarian Cookbook, Oil-Free* (Alabama: Thrash Publications, 1978), 182.

6. Ellis, F., et. al., "Incidence of Osteoporosis in Vegetarians and Omnivores," *American Journal of Clinical Nutrition* 1974; 27: 916.

7. Messina, V., Melina, V., Mangels, A.R., "A new food guide for North American Vegetarians," *Journal of the American Dietetic Association* 2003; 103: 771–75.

8. Mazess, R., "Bone mineral content of North Alaskan Eskimos," *American Journal of Clinical Nutrition* 1974; 27: 916–925.

9. McDougall, *The McDougall Program*, 384.

10. Lewinnek, G., "The significance and a comparative analysis of the epidemiology of hip fractures," *Clinical Orthopedic Related Research* 1980; 152: 35, cited in Klaper, Michael., M.D., *Pregnancy, Children, and the Vegan Diet* (Kapa'au, Hawaii: Gentle World, Inc., 1994), 16.

11. Parke, A. L., Hughes, G. R., "Rheumatoid Arthritis and Food: A Case Study," *British Medical Journal* (Clin Res Ed) June 20, 1981; 282(6281): 2027–2029.

"The case against heated milk protein," *Atherosclerosis* January–February 1971; 13: 137–139, and "Further evidence in the case against heated milk protein," *Atherosclerosis* January–February, 1972; 15: 129.

"Milk protein and other food antigens in atheroma and coronary heart disease," *American Heart Journal* February 1971; 81: 189.

12. Klaper, *Pregnancy, Children, and the Vegan Diet,* 41–42.

Ferrer, J. "Milk of dairy cows frequently contains a leukemogenic virus," *Science* 1981; 213: 1014–1015.

13. Mead Johnson Nutritionals, *Enfamil Family of Formulas: Expressing & Storing Breastmilk* (Indiana: Mead Johnson & Co.: 1996, 1997), 16.

14. Korenblat, P., "Immune responses of human adults after oral and parenteral exposure to bovine serum albumin," *Journal of Allergy* 1968; 41: 226.

"Unrecognized disorders frequently occurring among infants and children from the ill effects of milk," *Southern Medical Journal* 1938; 31: 1016.

Lindahl, O. "Vegan regimen with reduced medication in the treatment of bronchial asthma," *Journal of Asthma* 1985; 22(1): 45–55.

15. Mangels, Reed, Ph.D., R.D., cited in *Vegetarian Journal* magazine, January–February 1998, Vol. 17, No. 1, 2.

16. Bahna, S. L., and Heiner, D. C., *Allergies to Milk* (New York: Grune and Stratton: 1980); Gerrard, J. W., Mackenzie, J. W. A., Goluboff, N., et al. "Cow's milk allergy; prevalence and manifestations in an unselected series of newborns," *Acta Paediatr. Scand.* 1973; Supplement 234; and Grybowski, J. D., "Gastrointestinal milk allergy in infants," *Pediatrics* 1967; 40: 354, cited in Klaper, *Pregnancy, Children, and the Vegan Diet,* 60 Ziegler, E. E., Fomon, S. J., Nelson, S. E., et al., "Cow milk feeding in infancy: further observations on blood loss from the gastrointestinal tract," *Journal of Pediatrics* 1990; 116: 11–18.

17. Clyne, P. S., and Kulczycki, A., "Human breast milk contains bovine IgG. Relationship to infant colic?" *Pediatrics* 1991; 87: 439–444, cited in Barnard, Neal, M.D., *Food for Life* (New York: Three Rivers Press, 1993), 153.

18. "Cow Antibodies Are Linked to Colic in Babies," *The New York Times,* March 30, 1991, and *Pediatrics,* April 1991, cited in Jack, Alex, *Let Food Be Thy Medicine* (Becket, MA: One Peaceful World Press, 1991), 104.

19. McDougall, *The McDougall Program,* 37.

20. The lactose consumption (L) / galactose-1-phosphate uridyl transferase (T) ratio (L/T) was highly significantly correlated for ovarian cancer risk, with lactose being a dietary risk factor and transferase a genetic risk factor for

ovarian cancer. Cramer, D., et al., "Galactose Consumption and Metabolism in Relation to the Risk of Ovarian Cancer," *Lancet* 1989; 2: 66–71.

21. Simoons, F. J., "A geographic approach to senile cataracts: possible links with milk consumption, lactase activity, and galactose metabolism," *Digestive Diseases and Sciences* 1982; 27(3): 257–264, and Couet, C., Jan, P., and Debry, G., "Lactose and cataract in humans: a review," *Journal of the American College of Nutrition*, 1991; 10(1): 79–86, cited in Barnard, *Food for Life*, 13–14.

22. Hegsted, M. "Urinary calcium and calcium balance in young men as affected by level of protein and phosphorus intake," *Journal of Nutrition* 1981; 111: 553.

    Linkswiler, H., "Calcium retention of young adult males as affected by level of protein and calcium intake," *New York Academy of Science* 1974; 36: 333.

    Mazess, R., "Bone mineral content of North Alaskan Eskimos," *American Journal of Clinical Nutrition* 1974; 27: 916–925.

23. McDougall, *The McDougall Program*, 384.

24. McDougall, John A., M.D., and Mary McDougall, *The New McDougall Cookbook* (New York: Penguin Group, 1993), 24.

25. "A Multiple Share of Myeloma," *Medical World News*, May 16, 1969; 23, and "What Causes Cancer on the Farm?" *Medical World News*, January 14, 1972; 39.

    Thrash, Agatha, M.D., *The Animal Connection* (Alabama: Yuchi Pines Institute, 1980), Chapter 5.

26. Medline, "Many Women Quit Hormones," Associated Press, Laura Neergaard, AP Medical Writer, Thursday, October 24, 2002.

27. McDougall, *The McDougall Program*, 383.

28. Pawlak, Laura, Ph.D., R.D., lecture on *Alternative Medicine: An Objective View* (Emeryville, CA: Institute for Natural Resources, 1998), Troy, Michigan, June 1998.

7

CANCER

OVER ONE MILLION AMERICANS ARE RECEIVING medical care for the 200 different diseases classified as cancer.[1] The American Cancer Society (ACS) reports that 553,091 Americans died of cancer in 2000, making cancer the number two cause of death (behind heart disease) in this country. The ACS has stated that a woman has a 1 in 3 chance of developing cancer in her lifetime, and a man has a 1 in 2 chance.[2]

Approximately half of the known types of cancer are incurable at any stage.[3] It is long past time for the focus of the "War on Cancer," declared by President Nixon back in 1971, to switch from "cure" to "prevention." Yet, according to the National Cancer Institute's cancer research portfolio for fiscal year 2002, only 493 of a total of 2238 funded clinical trials and projects were categorized as "prevention."[4] This category includes money spent on the education and training of investigators, and research on vaccines and chemoprevention. Between 1940 and 1990, the death rates from the six most common cancers either increased or remained the same.[5] Further, between 1973 and 1999, American cancer death rates for all sites combined either increased or remained the same.[6]

Around 400 B.C.E., Hippocrates referred to the distended veins radiating from a breast tumor as being like the limbs of a crab—*karkinoma* in Greek. Our term "cancer" comes from the Latin. In the 1960s, the etiology was discovered in the mutation of genes, which can result in the production of a malfunctioning or non-functioning protein. Although mutations occur every day on a random basis, especially when our cells are saturated with carcinogens like pollution, contaminants, and radiation, few of these mutations are cancer-related. A cancer cell evolves when a mutation, usually due to injury caused by smoking, radiation, or toxic chemicals, causes genes that should be dormant to begin to produce enzymes involved in cancer development (proto-oncogenes).

The cell containing the mutated gene will divide in about 100 days. The new cancer genes, called oncogenes, produce abnormal proteins that are necessary for the cancer cell's destructive work. If normal and healthy suppressor genes (which typically control the growth and division of cells) are also mutated, the cancerous oncogene cells will continue to divide wildly. This is called cloning, and it results in a mass of identical cells called a tumor. Unlike normal cells, which are programmed for cell death, oncogenes do not contain signals to stop or control their growth. Further, the metabolism of a cancer cell is more flexible than that of healthy cells, in that many cancer cells do not require oxygen to continue. After a year, there will be twelve or more cells, which form a cancer; after six years, the cancerous lump will consist of about a million cells, measuring about a millimeter in size. In 90% of cases, the cells also will have entered the bloodstream and spread, in a process called metastasis.[7]

More and more physicians and researchers studying the etiology of cancer say that over 80% of cancers are attributable to factors we can potentially control,[8] and that 50–80% of all cancers include poor nutrition as a significant risk factor.[9] As doctors today begin to realize that 80–90% of all cancers are self-inflicted, often unknowingly (because of the dismal efforts of our government and its tax-funded agencies to better educate citizens based upon existing international data), they see that we make choices every day that can lead to cancer. For example, we may ingest chemicals and hormones of all types (primarily or secondarily, e.g., by eating animal flesh grown with these contaminants), utilize tobacco products, fail to exercise, or practice other poor habits. Table 7 illustrates the factors related to the development of cancer.

This information is now corroborated by the National Academy of Sciences, the U.S. Department of Health and Human Services, the National Cancer Institute, and the

TABLE 7.
ESTIMATED PERCENTAGES OF CANCER
DUE TO SELECTED FACTORS[10]

Factor	Estimated Percentage
Diet	35%–60%
Tobacco	30%
Alcohol	3%
Radiation	3.00%
Medications	2%
Air and water pollution	1–5%

Reprinted from Barnard, Neal, M.D., *Food for Life* (New York: Three Rivers Press, 1993), 60, by permission of Neal Barnard, M.D.

American Cancer Society. Research shows that diet and nutrition are factors in 60% of women's cancers and 40% of men's cancers, and that tobacco usage is a factor in about 30% of human cancers.[11] As far back as 1892, *Scientific American* magazine printed the observation, "[C]ancer is most frequent among those branches of the human race where carnivorous habits prevail."[12] One hundred years later, the American Cancer Society announced, "Some scientists believe that Americans could eliminate 80–100% of lung cancer, 90% of colon cancer, and more than 75% of breast and prostate cancers *if* they adopt the lifestyle and diet of countries with the lowest rates of these diseases."[13] Unfortunately, not many have heeded the call.

Nutrition plays a vital role in the prevention or development of cancer, as I shall demonstrate below in the discussion of key factors such as immune system strength and the effects of protein, fat, hormones, and phytonutrients.

• IMMUNE SYSTEM

There is a clear cause-and-effect relationship between nutrition, immunity, and cancer, and with each decade of life, the immune system needs a greater boost from nutrition.[14] In 1995, *Nutrition Digest* stated, "Nutrition alters the expression of genes involved in the development of cancer."[15] Cancer can actually develop as a result of poor nutrition, which can damage genetic material, or repair its structure abnormally. Poor nutrition is also one of the most frequent reasons that the immune system malfunctions.

The immune system is a complex interaction of blood cells, proteins, and processes that defend the body against infection, foreign substances, and cancer cells that develop spontaneously in the body. Two of the major armies of the immune system are white blood cells and antibodies, which are made from white blood cells called plasma cells. These armies arise separately but are related and dependent upon each other for their development and maturity. Another important type of white blood cell, the lymphocyte, is classified as a B-cell or a T-cell, based on outer markings of the surface membrane. A third component of the white blood cell groupings are the phagocytes, which "patrol" for invaders.[16]

In a healthy immune response, blood cells originating mainly from the thymus gland (T-cells) are the soldiers ready to attack and destroy. Their receptors attach directly onto surface antigens of any foreign cell. The B-cells secrete proteins called antibodies that are shaped to attach to antigens (foreign invader molecules) as well. Like arrows embedded in the center of a target, antibodies tag foreign cells, including precancer cells, for the "kill" by other members of the immune system. Additional cells called natural killer cells also originate in the bone marrow and emit chemicals that may lead the precancer cell to self-destruct.

Improper nutrition negatively affects all components of the immune system, including T-cell function, other cellular-related killing, B-cells' ability to make antibodies, the functioning of the complement proteins (as in inflammation during immune response), and phagocytic function. When these abilities are impaired, the immune system's capacity to identify, tag, scavenge, and eliminate foreign invaders such as cancer is greatly diminished. If a cancerous cell is allowed by a compromised immune system to hide, feed, and spread, its host has become a cancer victim.[17]

The German Cancer Research Center in Heidelberg has been comparing vegetarians to nonvegetarians since 1978. When they measured the white blood cells of each group, they found that the vegetarians had more than double the ability of nonvegetarians to destroy cancer cells.[18] While some current studies show varying results for vegetarians, it is recommended that future studies clarify a nutrient-dense and health-promoting plant-based diet, versus a diet that is meat-free but contains plenty of junk food and refined foods, for accurate results and conclusions. In 1995, the *Journal of the National Cancer Institute* clearly stated, "High-fat diets suppress the immune response."[19] In 1995, the Nutrition Action Health Letter reported that women who ate fruit about six times a day had a 35% lower risk of breast cancer than women who ate fruit only once a day, and that women who reported eating an average of five servings of vegetables a day had a 46% lower risk of breast cancer than women who ate only one or two servings per day.[20] And a study of colon cancer in nurses, directed by Dr. Walter Willett, a professor at Harvard University, followed 88,751 nurses over ten years and ultimately recommended, "The less red meat the better. . . . At most, it should be eaten only occasionally. . . . It may be maximally effective not to eat red meat at all."[21]

• PROTEIN AND FAT

Animal proteins such as casein, found in cow-milk products, have been linked to many different forms of cancer. One study cites the correlation between increased dietary intake

of animal proteins and an increased incidence of breast cancer.[22] Another found that breast cancer strikes American
women four times more often than Japanese women.[23]
Further, when Japanese women do get breast cancer, they
tend to survive longer—and this is independent of age, tumor
size, estrogen receptor status, extent of spread to lymph
nodes, and microscopic appearance of cancer cells.[24] It is this
author's conclusion that lifestyle factors including diet and
exercise are again the main protective factors.

In a study conducted in Sweden, 60,000 women aged 40
to 76 with no diagnosis of cancer were asked to complete a
67-item food frequency questionnaire. During the 4.2-year
follow-up, 674 women developed invasive breast cancer.
Statistical calculations by the investigators revealed that an
increased consumption of monounsaturated fat (found in
olive oil and canola oil) was associated with significantly
decreased risk for invasive breast cancer, whereas consumption of polyunsaturated fat (found in fish and some vegetable
oil) was associated with significantly increased risk.[25] Note,
however, cautions concerning excessive fat intake of *any*
kind, which continues to raise the risks of obesity and its
related diseases.

The Canadian Diet and Breast Cancer Prevention Study
Group looked at 800 women separated into two groups: one
consumed a 20% fat diet, the other a 32% fat diet. All of
these women were at risk for breast cancer. Over a two-year
period, the women consuming the 20% fat diet experienced
a greater reduction in dense breast tissue, which has been
associated with increased breast cancer risk. Women who
lost weight also experienced a decrease in the density of their

breast tissue. Another interesting finding was that the women on the 20% fat diet also experienced a 20% decrease in blood estrogen levels, which may be related to the tissue density reduction.[26]

For a woman who has breast cancer that has spread to other parts of the body, the risk of dying from the disease at any point in time increases 40% for every 1,000 grams of fat consumed monthly.[27] Research done in Italy and France concluded that women with breast cancer tended to consume considerably more cow milk, high-fat cheese, and butter than healthy women of the same age.[28] Soy, however, has been shown to help reduce the incidence of breast cancer.[29]

• HORMONES

Diet has a significant effect on the hormones that affect breast cancer risk, such as estrogen. High dietary fat levels artificially elevate hormone levels, causing overstimulation of the mammary tissues, and repeated bouts of this inflammation cause scarring and plugged milk ducts, which form cysts, an associated precursor to breast cancer.[30] High fat levels also provide a favorable home for anaerobic bacteria, which create estrogens from the bile that stimulates growth in sex organs, as well as carcinogenic substances such as deoxycholic acid, at a significantly higher rate.[31] On a vegetarian diet, breast cells have less exposure to estrogen, and therefore a reduced cancer risk.

As ovaries produce estrogen (in its conjugated form) and release it into the blood, the liver dumps the hormone into the intestine as part of fecal waste. According to Gail McIntyre, M.D., when conjugated estrogen comes into contact with the products of a low-fiber, high-animal-protein diet, bacteria are produced that make the beta-glucuronidase enzyme. This enzyme deconjugates the estrogen, which now passes from the digestive system back into the bloodstream, returning to the body and breast. Dr. McIntyre further notes that we can reduce the excess estrogen by eating lower-glycemic foods and thus decreasing the amount of insulin our bodies release when we eat. Fiber helps by increasing the fecal loss of estrogen, thereby lowering blood estrogen levels. And vegetarians, as we have established, consume large amounts of fiber-rich plant food. One study concluded that women who took in only one-third as much animal protein and fat excreted two to three times as much estrogen. Another study cited in the *New England Journal of Medicine* specifically noted the lower concentration of estrogens circulating in vegetarians. These findings suggest that vegetarian women are processing estrogen differently than non-vegetarian women, and can eliminate it more quickly from the body.

Insulin and testosterone levels are also implicated in hormonally triggering breast tissue problems, and, like estrogen, are influenced tremendously by obesity and dietary fat.[32] Exercise as well as diet can help maintain appropriate fat and hormone levels; recent research cited in the *New England Journal of Medicine* concluded that just four hours of exercise per week can reduce blood estrogen levels and cut breast cancer by 36–72%.[33]

In 1982, the National Academy of Sciences issued a 472-page report called *Diet, Nutrition, and Cancer.* In the panel's final review of hundreds of current medical studies, it concluded that the "modern" diet—high in saturated fat, animal protein, sugar, and chemical additives—was associated with a majority of cancers, including malignancies of the breast, colon, lung, prostate, uterus, esophagus, and stomach. The report noted that although the Academy had traditionally expected pathology to develop from a lack of nutrients, they now recognized that certain problems were associated with an "abundant and apparently normal" diet. The report called for substantial decreases in meat, poultry, egg, dairy, and refined carbohydrates. It also recommended increased intake of whole cereal grains, vegetables, and fruits. Finally, the report stated, "The dietary changes now underway appear to be reducing our dependence on foods from animal sources."[34]

In 1984, the American Cancer Society published its first dietary guidelines in respect to the cause and prevention of cancer. Although its recommendations were weak, in light of the mountains of evidence supporting the fact that diet is a major factor in many cancers, it did recommend increased fiber and vegetables, and vitamins A and C, and a decrease in total fat, alcoholic beverages, and salt-cured, smoked, and nitrite-cured meats. It also warned against obesity.[35] Later revised guidelines specifically recommend a plant-based diet, choosing whole grains over refined carbohydrates, and a limited intake of fat, especially animal fat.[36] Further, the number one recommendation of the World Cancer Research Fund and American Institute for Cancer Research in their 1997 report was: "Choose predominantly plant-based diets rich in a variety of vegetables and fruits, legumes, and minimally processed starchy staple foods."[37]

The China Health Study, a comprehensive epidemiological study conducted in the 1990s, sponsored by the U.S. National Cancer Institute and the Chinese Institute of Nutrition and Food Hygiene, and run by medical expert and biochemist T. Colin Campbell of Cornell University, correlated nutrient intakes and disease mortality rates in sixty-five rural Chinese counties. Less than 1% of deaths were caused by coronary artery disease, and breast cancer, colon cancer, lung cancer, and other malignancies commonly found in the West were comparatively rare. Table 8 highlights only some of the many statistically significant findings of the study.

Important conclusions drawn by the researchers were as follows:

- Fat consumption should be reduced to 10–15% of total calories
- A variety of fresh plant foods in the diet translates to the lowest risk for cancer.
- Eating animal protein is linked with chronic disease. (Chinese typically derive 11% of their calories from animal protein; the typical American obtains 70% of his or her calories from animal protein). Further, meat consumption is not needed to prevent iron-deficiency anemia; the Chinese plant-based diet was found to be sufficiently rich in iron for good health.
- The typical "rich" American diet promotes early menstruation, and may increase the risk of breast and reproductive organ cancer.
- Cow-milk products are not needed to prevent osteoporosis.

TABLE 8.
FIVE MEASURES OF COMPARISON
FROM THE CHINA HEALTH STUDY

Measure	Chinese	American
Dietary fiber (grams/day)	33.3	11.1
Plant protein (% daily protein intake)	89	30
Dietary fat (% of total calories)	14.5	38.8
Dietary calcium (mg/day)	544	1143
Blood plasma cholesterol (mg/dl)	127	212

Dr. Campbell summarizes that the Chinese realize that "animal-based agriculture is not the way to go."[38]

Researchers at the Fox Chase Cancer Center in Philadelphia reviewed thirty-seven studies, involving 10,000 people in fifteen different countries. They reported that those who ate a diet high in whole grains and other plant foods had about 40% less risk of colorectal cancer.[39] David Heber, M.D., Ph.D., of UCLA's Clinical Nutrition Division points out that, "Around the world, diets low in fruits, vegetables, and soy protein have higher rates of prostate cancer."[40] And Seventh Day Adventists, a religious group that is mainly vegetarian, have a very low incidence rate of cancer and cardiovascular disease when compared to nonvegetarians.[41]

The chief surgeon of the National Cancer Institute, Dr. Steven A. Rosenberg, who operated on President Ronald Reagan's colon cancer in 1985, prescribed a modified whole-grain diet for Reagan, rather than chemotherapy or radiation treatment.[42] Grains have been linked to reduction of colon cancer (in comparison studies involving Finnish diets high in fiber)[43] and of many other cancers—yet the average American eats only one serving of a whole grain per week.[44] Interestingly, in that same year Dr. Rosenberg published a report with the Institute, stating that "except possibly in selected patients with cancer of the stomach, there has been no demonstrated improvement in the survival of patients with the ten most common cancers when radiation therapy, chemotherapy, or both have been added to surgical resection." (The ten most common cancers as cited in this report were those involving the lung, prostate, breast, uterus, colorectum, bladder, pancreas, stomach, skin, and kidneys.) Here is a list of common treatments for cancer that have been suspected of actually decreasing survival by lowering the body's immune defenses against cancer:

- major surgery
- blood transfusion
- radiation
- chemotherapy
- lymph node irradiation
- lymph node removal
- high-fat diet (exemplified by the meals served in almost all American hospitals)

While it has been proven that vegetarians do have less cancer than omnivores, some studies note that there are usually several differences in the lifestyles between the two. Vegetarians are less likely to be obese, exercise more, go for more medical check-ups, and smoke less than the general population. While the average Westerner eats 15 grams of fiber a day (our National Cancer Institute recommends 20–35), the average vegetarian eats 30–45 grams per day. Not only do vegetarians eat more phytochemicals and antioxidants than nonvegetarians, but it has also been found that lacto-ovo vegetarian diets are about 10% lower in fat calories than the SAD, while vegan diets are usually 20% lower.[45]

If we begin to see that there are several prerequisites for the development of cancer, then the typical American view that cancer "just comes with age" becomes much less bleak. For example, there are five separate mutation stages that must occur for a cell to become cancerous. While genetics play a role, and could, so to speak, start a person off at the second stage, the determining factors are likely to be the strength of the immune system and the healthfulness of the environment—both of which can be severely undermined by improper diet. Below, we will look at the digestive system as an example of how a systemic weakness can develop and allow the progression of cancer.

A healthy digestive system in a human adult would normally eliminate solid waste approximately two to three times a day, and urinate about four to six times a day. The more that is eaten or drunk, the more frequent the elimination. The stool should be moderately soft and easy to pass without strain, physical effort, tension, or pain. If it accumulates between eliminations to the point where intestinal bloating and discomfort occur, or if it is difficult to pass, it is not a healthy stool, and it can contribute to various disease processes, including cancer. This is where plant fiber is so important. The fiber provides the bulk necessary for the intestinal muscle to "pull" the waste out efficiently. Unlike refined flours and sugars, animal products, alcohol, and fats, which do not provide bulk, plant fiber comes in a variety of refined carbohydrates. Once all soluble nutrients are derived from the foods in the human digestive system, the indigestible fibers mix with the "friendly" bacteria and organisms, and hold water to form the bulk of the stool.[46]

A normal stomach can empty after three to 4.5 hours. Saliva is produced on regular mealtime schedules, when normal eating patterns are established by the individual. The salivary glands become filled with amylase in order to digest carbohydrates with the greatest potency when food is expected. If food is taken ahead of time (or even chewing gum before meals), amylase is not yet made, and digestion will not be as efficient. There is a trickle-down effect onto each organ of the digestive system, as it is now being asked to perform a task on a substance that has not been properly prepared for it to do its task. Overeating can cause digestive overload, resulting in undesired effects in gastric juices, bile, and the organs and glands themselves. It promotes partial digestion and the production of aldehydes, amines, alcohols, esters, and other toxic substances from fermentation, causing a higher level of toxins to accumulate in the blood.

Looking at simple "heartburn/indigestion" will serve as an example of an early warning system that the body is not functioning properly. The stomach manufactures hydrochloric acid in order to digest the food it is sent. If there is not enough of this acid, the food simply rots in the moist, dark, 98.6°F atmosphere. The balance of hydrochloric acid will be insufficient if the food is of a type not easily digested by the human body. The stomach muscle will try to churn harder, in order to bring the food into contact with the acid. At some point, fermentation begins, producing other deviant organic acids as a byproduct. The stomach continues to churn at an accelerated rate, and some of these deviant acids (sometimes mixed with the offending foods and the hydrochloric acid) are regurgitated into the esophagus. When the epithelial lining stings, people say they have "heartburn," and often they take an antacid. The symptom disappears, as the acids (including the needed hydrochloric acid) are neutralized. However, now the stomach's job has been thwarted, and the rest of the digestive tract suffers as this fermenting, undigested food moves through, potentially overstressing the liver and pancreas in the effort to complete the digestive process of these inappropriate foods. These stresses compound over time, and, in an environment filled with free radicals, the system is weakened and made vulnerable to the onset of cancer and other degenerative disease.

Colitis (irritation and inflammation of the large intestinc/colon) is usually "treated" with laxatives, antispasmodics, bulk agents, tranquilizers, sedatives, anti-diarrhea medications, diets high in cow-milk dairy products and low in fiber, and trips to a mental health professional to learn to handle stress. The truly effective treatment, however, is a diet free of animal products and high in fiber from natural plant food sources. Sometimes specific foods need to be eliminated for reasons of individual allergic response. When the bowel contents are changed, the bowel behavior is changed.[47]

A study published in the *Scandinavian Journal of Gastroenterology* concluded that the fewer cruciferous vegetables consumed, the greater the risk for colon polyps, and the larger and more abnormal the polyps.[48] Cruciferous vegetables include Brussels sprouts, cauliflower, kale, kohlrabi, rutabaga, turnips, mustard, and other greens. Researchers in South Africa have associated hemorrhoids with high-fat, low-fiber diets,[49] and concluded that the absence of hiatus hernia among Ugandans was due to their high-fiber, plant-based diet. The scientists suggested that the main cause of colon polyps and hiatus hernia (which can be precursors to cancer) is eating meat and other foods that increase intra-abdominal pressure as the body tries to eliminate stools that are lower-weight, harder, and more compacted than normal, with an average transit time in the bowels double that of people not eating the offending foods.[50] In addition, British researchers have concluded that eating white flour, refined sugar, and other refined carbohydrates reduces fecal bulk, allowing intense bowel muscle spasms to occur. This type of dietary intake has been associated with ulcerative colitis, non-occlusive ischemic colitis, diverticular disease and irritable bowel syndrome.[51]

Some pre-cancers that develop over time are associated with deficiencies in particular vitamins. Cervical dysplasia is a premalignant lesion of the uterine cervix and is associated with an increased risk of cervical cancer. Research has linked cervical dysplasia not only to low blood levels of vitamin C, but also to low blood levels of beta carotene. In one study, the severity of the disease was observed to increase as beta carotene blood levels decreased.[52]

Several phytonutrients that can prevent and treat cancer have been identified in fruits and vegetables. Among them are citrus fruits (e.g., oranges, lemons, limes), which contain liminoids. Liminoids stimulate the production of enzymes assumed to assist in cancer prevention in the lung and other areas. Grapefruits, specifically, contain a type of fiber that may help reduce cholesterol. The red-orange fruits and vegetables (like carrots, red peppers, raspberries, cantaloupe, papaya, watermelon, mango, and red grapefruit) contain high contents of carotenoids, which have been shown to boost immunity and reduce the risk of heart disease and cancer, cell damage, and other age-related disorders. Lycopene, another carotenoid, is found in high concentrations in tomatoes, and can prevent colon, rectal, and stomach cancers. It has also been shown to slow the growth of existing cancers, and to prevent macular degeneration—which is the leading cause of blindness among older Americans. Sulforaphane and indoles (which become more bioavailable once cooked) are found especially in broccoli, cabbage, bok choy, and other vegetables. These two phytonutrients help in the prevention of cancer, especially colon cancer.[53]

Plant families that have been scientifically identified to work against cancer include *umbelliferae*, resembling umbrellas (carrots, parsnips, celery, parsley, cilantro); *cucurbitaceae*, with long vines (pumpkins, cucumbers, squash, melon); citrus from the *rutaceae* family (lemons, citrons, oranges, tangerines, grapefruit, mandarin oranges); and the *solanaceae* family (tomatoes, eggplant, peppers).

The following natural foods have also been found to have cancer-fighting properties: flax seeds, olives, avocados, soy, green peas, wheat germ (the embryo of the wheat seed) and whole wheat grain, broccoli, spinach, strawberries, grapes, green tea, garlic, and onion.[54]

The vitamins and phytonutrients in plants work to defend our bodies against free radicals, which play a major role in the development of cancer. A free radical is a molecule that has an unpaired electron in its orbit. This makes the molecule unstable, like a wheel out of round. It causes the molecule to react with other molecules at the wrong time and place, as it constantly tries to stabilize itself. Radiation sickness is one example of how free radical activity works in the human body. Antioxidants are molecules that seem designed to reinstate the free radical to electron balance. They work to stop free radicals from harming healthy cells and slow the process of precancer turning to cancer. They also may be able to slow the formation of tumors.[55] Human enzymes (proteins that enhance chemical reactions or conversions) thought to be formed in the spleen, such as super oxide dismutase and catalase, are examples of endogenous antioxidants. They convert free radicals into harmless waste products easily eliminated through the kidneys.

Phytochemicals found in plant foods actually help to reinstate these antioxidants to their protective activities. Specifically, flavonoids, phenolic acids, glucarates, carotenoids, and coumarins serve as attack molecules of sorts, while triterpenes and phytosterols suppress free radicals and slow the process of cancer. Vitamin E is an antioxidant, reinstating free radicals to an electron balance.[56] Vitamin A can also stimulate the body's defenses against disease by increasing the size of the thymus, which is vital to the cells' protection but tends to shrink when the body is subjected to stress, including disease and malnutrition.[57]

In research conducted on 9,959 cancer-free Finnish men and women aged 15 to 99 years, flavonoids were studied in their relationship to cancer. Dietary histories were obtained, and a follow-up was conducted from 1967 to 1991. During the follow-up, 997 cancer cases and 151 lung cases were diagnosed. An inverse association was observed between the intake of flavonoids and the incidence of all cites of cancer combined.[58] The author wishes to point out that, while there are over 20,000 identified flavonoids in nature, whole food sources are preferable to supplements. This also holds true for many other nutrients, including carotenoids, of which over 300 have been identified nature. At least thirty different carotenoids are active in a human cell.[59]

It is prudent to avoid foods that can help produce free radicals. The omega-3 fatty acids from fish, unlike the more stable omega-3's found in plant foods, are highly unstable molecules and tend to decompose, unleashing free radicals.[60] Although most vegetable fats and oils will not elevate cholesterol levels, coconut and palm kernel oils are exceptions and should be eliminated or kept to a minimum. Polyunsaturated fats reacting with oxygen or enzymes produce free radicals and hydroperoxides, which can damage cell membranes and contribute to the development of cancer. As stated earlier, monounsaturated fats like olive oil and canola oil have been shown to have a protective effect against cancer.

Interestingly, excess iron absorbed primarily from animal sources is a perfect catalyst for free radical formation—unlike the iron in plant foods, which is limited better by the body's natural metabolism. While researchers have come to various conclusions regarding excess iron storage, one study published on 2,000 men in Finland in 1992 concluded that the more iron stored in the body, the higher the risk for heart disease.[61] Unfortunately, except in those who are menstruating or who donate blood, the human body has no way of ridding itself of excess iron, but simply continues to store it. Dr. Randall B. Lauffer, a biochemist at Harvard University, has identified iron as a key component of the free radical theory of disease. He recommends a "push toward a more vegetarian-style diet . . . ."[62]

The intake of many different kinds of plant foods is higher in those persons found to be at a lower risk of cancer.[63] The evidence is clear: people who regularly eat substantially more plant foods are far less likely to succumb to a huge range of cancers.[64]

1. McDougall, John A., M.D., *The McDougall Program* (New York: Penguin Group, 1990), 314.
2. American Cancer Society, "Cancer Statistics Slide Set 2003," http://www.cancer.org/docroot/PRO_1_1_Cancer_Statistics_2002_slides.zip.asp?sitearea=PRO.
3. Wagman, Richard, M.D., F.A.C.P., ed., *The New Complete Medical and Health Encyclopedia, Vol. 2* (Chicago: J. G. Ferguson Publishing Company, 1987), 559–561.
4. National Cancer Institute, "Cancer Research Portfolio," http://research-portfolio.cancer.gov/prevention.html.
5. McDougall, *The McDougall Program,* 314.
6. National Cancer Institute, Division of Cancer Control and Population Sciences, "Surveillance, Epidemiology, and End Results Program, 1973–1999" (National Cancer Institute, 2002), cited in American Cancer Society, "Cancer Statistics Slide Set 2003."

7. McDougall, *The McDougall Program,* 314–315.

8. Barnard, Neal, M.D., *Food for Life* (New York: Three Rivers Press, 1993), xi.

9. Quillin, 1994, cited in Pawlak, Laura, Ph.D., R.D., *A Perfect 10: Phyto "New-trients" against Cancers* (Emeryville, CA: Biomed General Corporation, 1998), 1.

10. National Cancer Institute, *Cancer Rates and Risks* (Washington D.C., 1985) and Doll, R., and Peto, R., "The Causes of Cancer: Quantitative Estimates of Avoidable Risks of Cancer in the United States Today," *Journal of the National Cancer Institute* 1981; 66: 1191–1308, cited in Barnard, *Food for Life,* 60.

11. Simone, Charles B., M.D., *Cancer and Nutrition* (New York: Avery Publishing Group, Inc., 1992), 3–4.

12. Barnard, *Food for Life,* 60.

13. Pawlak, *A Perfect 10,* 144.

14. Chandra, R., "Nutrition and the immune system: an introduction," *American Journal of Clinical Nutrition* 1997; 66(2): 460S–463S, cited in Pawlak, *A Perfect 10,* 16.

15. Pawlak, *A Perfect 10,* 21.

16. Simone, *Cancer and Nutrition,* 43–45.

17. Pawlak, *A Perfect 10,* 8–15.

18. Barnard, *Food for Life,* 78.

19. *Journal of the National Cancer Institute* (1995), cited in Pawlak, *A Perfect 10,* 38.

20. *Nutrition Action Health Letter* (1995), cited in Pawlak, *A Perfect 10,* 155.

21. Willett, Walter C., et al., "Relation of Meat, Fat, and Fiber Intake to the Risk of Colon Cancer in a Prospective Study Among Women," *New England Journal of Medicine* 1990; 323: 1664–1672, and Toufexis, A., "Red Alert on Red Meat," *Time* magazine, December 24, 1990.

22. Nixon, Daniel M., M.D., and Alison Brown, *The Cancer Recovery Eating Plan* (New York: Cerier Book Development, Inc., 1994/1996), 32–33.

23. Pawlak, *A Perfect 10,* 24.

24. Wynder, E. L., Kajitani, T., Kuno, J., Lucas, J. C. Jr., DePalo, A., and Farrow, J., "A comparison of survival rates between American and Japanese patients with breast cancer," *Surgery, Gynecology and Obstetrics,* 1963; 117: 196–200; and Gregorio, D. I., Emrich, L. J., Graham, S., Marshall, J. R., and Nemoto, T., "Dietary fat consumption and survival among women

with breast cancer," *Journal of the National Cancer Institute*, 1985; 254: 2728, cited in Barnard, *Food for Life,* 79.

25. *Archives of Internal Medicine* 1998; 158: 41–45, cited in Hosford, C., ed., "Medical Updates—Monounsaturated Fats Cut Breast Cancer Risk," in *Life Extension* magazine, Vol. 4, No. 7, 24.

26. *Journal of the National Cancer Institute,* 1997; 89: 488, cited in "Findings," *Loma Linda University Vegetarian Nutrition & Health Newsletter* 1997, Vol. 1, No. 1, 5.

27. Gregorio, D. I., Emrich, L. J., Graham, S., Marshall, J. R., and Nemoto, T., "Dietary fat consumption and survival among women with breast cancer," *Journal of the National Cancer Institute*, 1985; 254: 2728.

28. Toniolo, Paolo, et al., "Calorie-providing nutrients and risk of breast cancer," *Journal of the National Cancer Institute* 1989; 81: 278–286.

29. Troll, W., "Blocking of Tumor Promotion by Protease Inhibitors," in Burchenal, J. H. and Oettgen, H. F., eds., *Cancer: Achievements, Challenges, and Prospects for the 1980s, Vol. 1* (New York: Grune and Stratton, 1980), 549–555.

30. McDougall, *The McDougall Program,* 359.

31. Pritikin, Nathan, and Patrick McGrady, *The Pritikin Program for Diet and Exercise* (New York: Grosset and Dunlap, Inc., 1979), 31.

32. Pawlak, *A Perfect 10,* 147.

33. Ibid., 149.

34. McDougall, John A., M.D., *McDougall's Medicine: A Challenging Second Opinion* (Clinton, NJ: New Win Publishing, Inc., 1985), 42.

35. *The American Medical Association Family Guide* (New York: Random House, 1987), cited in Jack, Alex, *Let Food Be Thy Medicine* (Becket, MA: One Peaceful World Press, 1991), 31–32.

36. American Cancer Society Web site: www.cancer.org.

37. World Cancer Research Fund and American Institute for Cancer Research, "Food, Nutrition and the Prevention of Cancer: a Global Perspective," 1997, p. 509.

38. Chen Junshi, T. Colin Campbell, Li Junyao, and Richard Peto, *Diet, Lifestyle, and Mortality in China* (New York: Cornell University Press, 1990); and Brody, Jane, "Huge Study of Diet Indicts Fat and Meat," *New York Times*, May 8, 1990, cited in Jack, *Let Food Be Thy Medicine*, 38–39.

39. Tock, B., Lanza, E., and Greenwald, P., "Dietary Fiber, Vegetables, and Colon Cancer: Critical Review and Meta-analyses of the Epidemiologic Evidence," *Journal of the National Cancer Institute* 1990; 82: 650–661.

40. Pawlak, *A Perfect 10*, 168.

41. Simone, *Cancer and Nutrition*, 37.

42. Rosenberg, Steven A., M.D., "Combined-modality therapy of cancer," *New England Journal of Medicine*; 312: 1512–1514, and Alex Jack, personal communication with the White House, July 1985, cited in Jack, *Let Food Be Thy Medicine*, 53–54.

43. Englyst, H. N., et al., "Nonstarch polysaccharide concentrations in four Scandinavian populations," *Nutrition and Cancer* 1982; 4: 50–60.

44. Pawlak, Laura, Ph.D., R.D., lecture on *Alternative Medicine: An Objective View* (Emeryville, CA: Institute for Natural Resources, 1998), Troy, Michigan, June 1998.

45. Weisberger, Ph.D., "How Vegetarian Diets Protect against Cancer," cited in *Loma Linda University Vegetarian Nutrition and Health Newsletter* 1997, Vol. 1, No. 1, 1–3.

46. McDougall, *The McDougall Program*, 330–332.

47. Ibid., 322–326.

48. Hoff, G., et al., *Scandinavian Journal of Gastroenterology* 1986; 21: 199, cited in Jack, *Let Food Be Thy Medicine*, 59.

49. Burkitt, D., "Varicose veins, deep vein thrombosis and hemorrhoids: epidemiology and suggested aetiology," *British Medical Journal* 1972; 2: 556.

50. Burkitt, D., and James, P., "Low-residue diets and hiatus hernia," *Lancet* 1973; 2: 128–130.

51. Grimes, D., "Refined carbohydrate, smooth-muscle spasm and disease of the colon," *Lancet* 1976; 1: 395–397.

52. Simone, *Cancer and Nutrition*, 97–98.

53. Barela, Sharon, ed., *Phyto-Rich Produce*, cited in *Veggie Life* magazine, July 1998, 57.

54. Pawlak, *A Perfect 10*, 28–30.

55. Ibid., 32–34.
Pawlak, Laura, Ph.D., R.D., lecture on *Alternative Medicine: An Objective View* (Emeryville, CA: Institute for Natural Resources, 1998), Troy, Michigan, June 1998.

56. Pawlak, *A Perfect 10*, 96.

57. Seifter, Eli, "A discussion of the relationship between vitamin A and the thymus," *Journal of Infectious Diseases* (September 1975), cited in Jensen, Bernard, M.D., and Mark Anderson, *Empty Harvest* (New York: Avery Publishing, 1990), 104.

58. Hosford, C., ed., "Medical Updates—Flavonoids and Cancer Risk," citing *American Journal of Epidemiology*, 1997; 146 (3): 223–230, in *Life Extension* magazine, 1998, Vol. 4, No. 7, 26.

59. Pawlak, *A Perfect 10*, 27.

60. Barnard, *Food for Life*, 9–10.

61. Salonen, J. T., Salonen, R., Nyyssonen, K., and Korpela, H., "Iron sufficiency is associated with hypertension and excess risk of myocardial infarction: the Kuopio Ischaemic Heart Disease Risk Factor Study (KIHD)," *Circulation* 1992; 85: 864.

62. Lauffer, R. B., *Iron Balance* (New York: St. Martin's Press, 1991), cited in Barnard, *Food for Life*, 11–12.

63. Wattenberg, L. W., et. al, *Cancer Prevention* (Boca Raton: CRC Press, 1992) 19–39.

64. *UC Berkeley Wellness Newsletter*, September 1997, cited in Pawlak, *A Perfect 10*, 143.

8

RELATED ETHICAL AND POLITICAL ISSUES

FOR THOSE WHO REMAIN SKEPTICAL THAT THE plant-based diet is ideal for humans because of what they have heard from other doctors or dietitians, I quote John McDougall, M.D.: "The burden of proof of the value of a therapy lies with those who recommend treatments that mutilate and debilitate the patient. The evidence that supports such therapies must show the benefits are greater than the side effects, including financial costs for the patient. In reality, therapics of unproved worth are now being prescribed and the burden of proof has been placed on those who question their worth."[1]

"Early detection" and "improved diagnostic technolo gy" may sound impressive, but these are techniques for identifying disease that is already present and active. I would rather my tax dollars went toward efforts to *prevent* me from having a chronic disease that would be "detectable" or "diagnosable." The slogan of Breast Cancer Awareness Month (whose chief sponsor is Zeneca Pharmaceuticals) says, "The best prevention is early detection." I believe this is inaccurate and misleading and should instead read, "The best prevention is health-promoting behavior." The *Berkeley Wellness Newsletter* (1997) states, "The real key to winning the war on cancer is not better treatment, but better prevention. Clearly this is the universal feeling of health professionals." The statement would be equally true if we replaced the word "cancer" with atherosclerosis, obesity, diabetes, or osteoporosis. Despite this, so little effort is made on the part of the American Medical Association to prevent disease that it is almost not worth mentioning.

The "germ theory" of disease was developed in the nineteenth century by Dr. Louis Pasteur. This philosophy, wherein germs invade and cause disease, can now be seen in more relative terms, with the research and technology now available to us. Germs are everywhere, and we are all exposed to them, but what is the difference between the person who "catches the cold" and the person who is resistant? A healthy constitution kept that way by proper living. If more than 200 viruses have been identified as the "cause" of the common cold, how efficient is it to have to identify and treat each individual virus, when strengthening the body is all that is necessary? Consider the illogic of this approach when there are almost 25,000 listed diseases known to date. However, our government and our country's physicians will not change their philosophy as long as there are multibillion-dollar industries promoting their diagnostics and pharmaceuticals, and lobbying comfortable officials.

Along with groups like the American Heart Association, which is connected to the government by strong financial ties, Washington tends to underfund crucial studies that could prove the superiority of a well-planned vegan diet with sufficient omega-3s and vitamin B12 over the SAD for optimal human health. Meanwhile, the government spends billions of taxpayer dollars on research and advertising campaigns that merely keep a number of bureaucrats on the payroll and the American population misinformed and sick. Through such programs as the National Beef Checkoff and dairy subsidies, the Department of Agriculture is required by law to promote agricultural commodities, even if they are at odds with your health.[2] Even the American Heart Association continues to serve beef, butter, cheese, and ice cream at its annual meetings and fundraisers! Imagine complimentary tobacco products and ashtrays at a meeting of the American Lung Association! Further, physicians continue to downplay the role of diet as disease prevention, in opposition to current research. Unfortunately, the education of physicians and their patients has a lot more to do with the advertising dollars spent by drug companies than with the use of preventive measures that would negate the need for these companies' products.

For example, at the 1998 International Conference on the Mediterranean Diet, organized by Oldways Preservation and Exchange Trust and the Harvard School of Public Health to study the effect of diet on heart disease, the following leading doctors and researchers dedicated to dietary prevention of chronic disease were *not* invited to participate in the forum: Dr. Dean Ornish, Dr. John McDougall, Cornell University's T. Colin Campbell, Dr. William Castelli of the Framingham Heart Study, Dr. William C. Roberts of the *American Journal of Cardiology*, Dr. Caldwell Esselstyn of the Cleveland Clinic, Dr. Charles Attwood (noted for his work with children and low-fat diets), and Patricia Bertron, R.D., of the Physicians' Committee for Responsible Medicine.

This absurdity would be analogous to holding a conference on the American presidential experience and not inviting Jimmy Carter, Gerald Ford, George Bush, Ronald Reagan, Bill Clinton, or George W. Bush. It is supposed by many of the leading proponents of low-fat diets in disease prevention that the exclusion was premeditated, because there was a political need to have the Mediterranean Diet approved by consensus at the Conference. The Conference ultimately stated its opinion that a healthful diet can be maintained without the limitation of fats to 30% or less, as long as calories are not excessive. However, note that most of the uninvited leaders in the field (mentioned above) favor limitation of fats to 10–15% of calories for chronic disease prevention. Perhaps input could have been gathered from these preventive medicine physicians toward a 100% plant-based "Mediterranean-style Diet" that would be naturally lower in saturated fat and cholesterol, and higher in fiber, than the original "Mediterranean Diet"!

In response to this conference, several of the excluded physicians and researchers were asked for their feedback for the Winter 1998 issue of *Vegetarian Voice* magazine. Some of these comments are listed below.

- Dr. Dean Ornish stated that the consensus from the Summit on Reversing Heart Disease, organized by the Cleveland Clinic in the fall of 1997, was that a low-fat vegetarian diet is optimal for most people. He noted the list of excluded guests to the Mediterranean diet conference and stated that, "While it may be easier to forge a consensus by excluding the scientific evidence from those who could present a different viewpoint, it seems unfortunate not to have all points of view represented. . . . I agree that one should reduce the intake of simple carbohydrates such as sugar, white flour, and alcohol, as well as hydrogenated and trans fatty acids. However, the [solution] is not to eat more fat, but to focus on a low-fat vegetarian diet based on whole foods and complex carbohydrates, such as fruits, vegetables, grains, and legumes (including soy products) in their natural states."

- Dr. T. Colin Campbell (of the China Study) noted, "Thirty-percent-fat diets should not even be regarded as low in fat. . . . For many people, a low-fat diet means 20–30% fat. . . . This is not what is meant by a healthy diet."

- Dr. John McDougall stated, "Hopefully, the next conference held to help the general public understand 'good nutrition' will focus on the 'best' diet for all people, rather than coming up with another compromise."

- Dr. Caldwell Esselstyn of the Summit on Cholesterol and Coronary Disease said, "My own preference is to tell the public the truth about the healthiest diet, and then let them decide what would be their degree of compliance."

- Dr. Attwood stated, "I am concerned about the animal protein excesses made available by frequent consumption of fish and low-fat dairy products.

Convincing studies have shown that excessive animal protein is a health risk independent of saturated fat."

- Patricia Bertron, R.D., the Staff Dietitian of the Physicians' Committee for Responsible Medicine, exclaimed, "How can this 'scientific group' suggest that . . . 'otherwise healthful diets need not limit fats to 30%, as current dietary guidance suggests, as long as these diets are not excessive in calories'?. . . . The definition of 'healthful diet' should be redefined as one based solely on whole grains, vegetables, fruits, and legumes. This is clearly the most beneficial diet of all."[3]

The U.S. government's dietary recommendations have influenced at least four generations of Americans, beginning with the Basic Four Food Groups in the 1950s. Parents who would give their own lives to save their children from a speeding car believe they are doing the right thing in feeding their children based on ADA guidelines. Yet, at the 2002 North American Vegetarian Society Conference, Dr. John McDougall spoke of the internal bodily "harm done with a fork and a knife" (the feeding of unhealthy foods) as analogous to a form of child abuse, by unknowing and sadly misled parents. The tragic result is that every child born in America today (and raised on the SAD) has a 1 in 3 chance of developing cancer and a 1 in 2 risk of developing heart disease, and 1 in every 8 of our girls will be stricken with breast cancer.

This chapter will take the discussion beyond these chronic diseases to examine some of the other problems related to the SAD—from early puberty to the destruction of planet Earth—that can be ameliorated by switching to the New Four Food Groups.

• HORMONES

As we saw earlier, high dietary fat levels artificially elevate hormone levels, and, while some research points to a protective effect against osteoporosis and heart disease, high levels of estrogens, particularly estradiol, have been implicated in breast cancer and abnormally early onset of puberty. The World Health Organization has been gathering statistics on the age of puberty worldwide for many years. In 1840, the average age of puberty in female humans was 17 years of age. Today, it is 12.5 years. The age of puberty is also dropping in England, Norway, Denmark, and Finland—other countries that eat the "western" diet.[4] Japan, as it slowly adopted the "western" diet, has had an accompanying drop in age of puberty from 15.2 years to 12.5 years, in the course of only 40 years.[5] Both African villages and the Chinese have retained many of their dietary traditions of eating plant-based foods, and they both average an onset of female puberty at 17 years of age.

Joanne Dorgan and some of her colleagues at the Fox Chase Cancer Center in Philadelphia recently tested 300 pre-pubescent girls, putting them on low-fat diets and then testing blood hormone levels over the years. The researchers were surprised that after five years, the girls on the diet had 29.8% lower levels of the hormone estradiol, 20.7% lower estrone levels, and 28.7% lower estrone sulfate levels during the first half of their menstrual cycles (all are variants of the hormone estrogen). The girls also had 27% higher levels of testosterone during the second half of their menstrual cycles compared with girls in the usual care group. After seven years, the progesterone levels of the girls in the diet group were 50% lower during the second half of their menstrual cycles than those of the girls in the usual care group. The researchers surmised that if the study had occurred earlier in the lives of these girls, their age of onset of menses and related risk of breast cancer in later life would have been lowered.

In addition to increasing the quantities of estrogens in the blood, high-fat animal products also take the place in the diet of needed plant foods, whose fiber helps the digestive system to enhance or control the circulating hormones. Vegetarians also produce more of estradiol's carrier protein, sex hormone binding globulin, which escorts the estrogens in an inactive state until they are actually needed.[6]

Researchers in the Netherlands conducted a study on sixty-three girls and their dietary intake that showed unequivocally that the girls who ate more vegetables and grains had less estradiol in their blood and later ages of onset of puberty.[7] Experts here in the U.S. became concerned about early puberty in girls after Marcia Herman-Giddens, a researcher at the University of North Carolina School of Public Health, published a study in 1997 of 17,000 American girls. By age eight, almost 50% of the black girls in the study, and about 15% of the white girls, had begun puberty (the source used "black" and "white" as indicators of ethnicity).

While research continues trying to decide whether the culprit of an abnormally early onset of puberty is the SAD's hormone load or its fat content, we are continually confronted with the problem of teen pregnancy. Regardless of mechanism, it is clear that educating our society to make the switch to a healthful vegan diet could result in decreased teen pregnancy rates and a reduction in many social and economic problems, rather than trying to pick up the pieces "when kids have kids."

In addition, this author posits that the hormones present naturally (and unnaturally, due to farming techniques) in animals used as food wreak havoc on the natural balance of hormones in the human body. Apparently, enough evidence already exists regarding the hormones routinely fed or implanted into the necks of cattle by American farmers— including estradiol, testosterone, progesterone, trenbolone acetate (synthetic testosterone) and zeranol (synthetic estrogen)—as the European Union (EU) has banned imports of American hormone-fed cattle since 1989.[8] In 1999, the United States complained to the World Trade Organization about the ban. The three-lawyer panel of the WTO ruled that the EU was required to pay $150 million per year as compensation for lost profit, despite the lengthy report by independent scientists showing that some hormones added to U.S. meat are "complete carcinogens" (capable of causing cancer by themselves). However, it was worth it to the European Union to pay $150 million per year to keep U.S. beef away from their citizens.[9]

According to John Robbins' groundbreaking book, *The Food Revolution,* more than 90% of U.S. cattle today receive hormone implants, and in the larger feedlots the figure is closer to 100%.[10] Although farming literature encourages farmers to use growth-stimulating implants routinely, it also warns that the implants can retard the development of the bull's reproductive organs, and that an improperly placed implant can create residues in the slaughtered animal.[11] There are several different types of implants available to farmers, and formula options change frequently. It is unlikely that most farmers have the time or expertise required to select the proper type, dose and frequency of administration for each animal.

• ANTIBIOTICS, PESTICIDES, AND GMOS

In addition to hormone implants, animals raised for food are given huge doses of antibiotics, which saturate their tissues, including their flesh and organs. But, as the Food and Drug Administration has acknowledged, antibiotics given to animals used for food may cause microbes to become resistant to drugs used to treat human illness: "Disease-causing microbes that have become resistant to drug therapy are an increasing public health problem. Tuberculosis, gonorrhea, malaria, and childhood ear infections are just a few of the diseases that have become hard to treat with antibiotic drugs. Part of the problem is that bacteria and other microorganisms that cause infections are remarkably resilient and can develop ways to survive drugs meant to kill or weaken them. This *antibiotic resistance*, also known as *antimicrobial resistance* or *drug resistance*, is due largely to the increasing use of antibiotics."

The author currently lives in a farming community and is shocked to hear farmer after farmer refer to the comparatively untreated livestock and plant crops that they grow separately from their other mass-produced and sold agricultural products, for their own family's use. It is not uncommon to hear, "I know what goes into those other animals (or onto those crops), and I'm not eatin' it!" Some of these objectionable crops may be "Roundup Ready" crops—genetically altered plant foods that are sprouted, then doused with the herbicide Roundup, so that anything and everything around the transgenic plants dies. The leaves of the altered crop foods are "burned," but apparently then begin to re-grow, while the soil, water, foliage, and animal balances are exterminated or damaged as far as the eye can see. Many farmers utilize these techniques on their 2,000-, 5,000-, or 10,000-acre (or more) farms, so this mass destruction goes on for miles and miles in America's farm lands.

Before delving deeper into the issue of pesticides, the author wishes to point out that Roundup Ready crops are not only destructive to the environment but also may be less nutritious than non-genetically engineered crops. For example, according to Monsanto's own tests, Roundup Ready soybeans contain 29% less of the brain nutrient choline, and 27% more trypsin inhibitor (a potential allergen that interferes with protein digestion), than normal soybeans. Soy products are often prescribed and consumed for their phytoestrogen content, but, according to the company's own tests, the genetically altered soybeans have lower levels of phenylalanine, an essential amino acid that affects levels of phytoestrogens. Levels of lectins, other fairly common allergens, are nearly double in the transgenic variety.[12]

The lack of information on the possible dangers of consuming genetically modified foods is a matter of deep concern to many scientists. Dr. Arpad Pusztai, senior scientist at the Rowett Research Institute in Aberdeen, Scotland, has published hundreds of scientific papers. His research with genetically modified potatoes gained him an interview with the major British television program *World In Action*. Dr. Pusztai's response to whether he would personally eat genetically modified potatoes was startling. "No, it is very, very unfair to use our fellow citizens as guinea pigs." Further, the *Lancet* describes the level of inaction by the FDA as, "astounding that FDA has not changed their stance on genetically modified food. . . . Governments should never have allowed these products into the food chain without insisting on rigorous testing for effects on health."[13]

There is also no research, to the knowledge of this author, that studies the cumulative effect of the synergistic combination of pesticides (over 300 are allowed by our Environmental Protection Agency!) within the human body. Insecticide use has increased tenfold since World War II, yet the USDA reports that crop loss due to insect damage has doubled in that same period. The fact is, chemicosterilants (insecticides and related man-made products) do not do the job their creators envisioned. Instead, they breed larger numbers of more resistant insects. (It is interesting to note that in 1989 in Indonesia, President Suharto banned at least fifty-seven organophosphate pesticides. He declared that the public rice fields had become more infested with predator pests, whose natural predators in nature had been killed by all of the chemicals.) Chemicosterilants are almost always carcinogenic to animals and humans, and they contaminate the water supply and destroy the soil's ecosystem. In short, these synthetic additives in farming have produced an agricultural system that is incompatible with the goal of producing healthy food crops.

Vegetarians and vegans receive far less exposure than meat eaters to synthetic environmental chemical contaminants like pesticides, hormones, and herbicides, because these substances are present in minimal amounts in the plants a human can eat in one day, compared to the amount that is concentrated in a piece of animal flesh after even a short lifetime's ingestion of thousands of pounds of contaminated food. An analysis of seventeen pesticides, toxins, and other chemical substances in the breast milk of vegetarian and nonvegetarian mothers found that except for equivalent ratings on polychlorinated biphenyls (PCBs), the highest vegetarian value was lower than the lowest value obtained in the nonvegetarian breast milk, and that the mean vegetarian levels were only 1–2% as high as the national average level of contaminants.[14]

Pesticides are associated with increased cancer rates, birth defects, developmental delays, endocrine dysfunction, reproductive problems, and other signs of neurotoxicity. These poisons are also killing off natural protective factors against candida albicans in humans (acidophilus bacilli, bifidus, etc.), which we need in order to combat complications arising from yeast infections. A diet high in refined carbohydrates and sugars worsens this problem exponentially. Finally, these chemical-contaminant cocktails can cause allergic symptoms that may appear in hundreds of different gastrointestinal, blood, immunity, respiratory, emotional, behavioral, and skin disorders. An allergy is sometimes called a "hypersensitivity"—literally an abnormal reaction by an overly sensitive individual. However, many preventive medicine practitioners are beginning to see these reactions as signals of environmental dangers that warrant the attention of all of us. Allergic symptoms have even been implicated in arthritis, lupus, asthma, sudden infant deaths, heart problems, and many other medical complications, including a growing number of behavioral and mental health disorders.

The United Nations has estimated that 2 million tons of pesticide applications are applied to our planet each year.[15]At this rate of 20 million tons each decade, what type of uncontrolled experiment are we conducting on our own survival? Beginning in 1989, the government of Sweden pledged to reduce pesticide use by 50% over five years. At the same time, our own government actually weakened restrictions on cancer-causing pesticides in foods. This meant that the existing weak standards on the 2.7 billion pounds of pesticides used annually here (75% of these pesticides are used directly in commercial agriculture, the remaining 25% are used on lawns) are actually worse than they were in 1989.

• BREEDING SUFFERING AND DISEASE

Despite the chemical arsenal we employ in our efforts to ensure that we are not eating diseased or contaminated foods, there are some diseases that remain a danger for those who continue to eat animals. The number one cause of bacterial food poisoning in the United States is the campylobacter germ. In one study, this germ was found in two-thirds of the chickens bought at stores around the country—yet the government does not require testing for it. Symptoms of campylobacter include diarrhea and fever lasting up to one week; the infection can also lead to Guillain-Barre syndrome and paralysis.[16] The Centers for Disease Control and Prevention estimate that of the 500 deaths per year from campylobacter, more than half are from contaminated poultry. The other two sources of campylobacter are unpasteurized cow milk and unchlorinated water. The study, which examined 1,000 chickens from thirty-six different cities, showed campylobacter in 63% of the birds and salmonella in 16%.

Some estimates of the presence of salmonella in chicken are as high as one in three. Salmonella causes "flu-like" symptoms, usually for several days. The Centers for Disease Control estimates the incidence rate to be between 400,000 and 4,000,000 every year (the range is wide to accommodate the many people who call it "the flu" and therefore are not recorded accurately). The main reason for the extent of the contamination is the assembly-line system of slaughter and processing. Chickens are raised by the thousands in small factories, living in accumulating feces for eight weeks; then their feathers are beaten off before their bodies are chopped up by the processing machinery at the plant. The bacteria growing in the feces, and in the birds' punctured intestines, are spread around before the dead birds are run through water and packaged for the store. The "chicken juice" in the package is actually water, blood, lymph, and feces.[17]

Approximately 8 billion chickens are raised annually in the U.S., de-beaked, and slaughtered after about seven to eight weeks of miserable life. The chickens raised as "broilers," bred for size and drastically overfed, grow so rapidly that they suffer from bone and muscle weaknesses, congestive heart failure, blindness, paralysis, brain damage, organ failure, and internal bleeding. Egg-laying hens are crowded into "battery cages," where they suffer severe feather loss, bruises and abrasions from rubbing against the wire, and where they cannot stretch their legs or wings or perform their normal behaviors. Seventy-five percent of U.S. hens used to lay eggs for human food are forced into molting through starvation for periods of ten to fourteen days at a time, and deprived of water for up to three days. The hens lose about 25% of their body weight in this horrific process designed to shock their bodies into a new laying cycle. The 300 million turkeys bred for food in the U.S. annually are products of artificial insemination, because, through so many generations of breeding for size, each turkey is too obese to be able to mate naturally.[18] Even if one feels no qualms about the cruelty of these production methods, how healthy can the hormones, pesticides, antibiotics, and adrenalized tissue (produced during the horror of confinement, transportation and slaughter) be for the human body?

In light of recent news stories about E. coli and other pathogens found in American beef, Farmed Animal Watch points out that common production practices, "whereby large numbers of animals are kept crowded together in manure, incubate a variety of hazardous pathogens." The group quotes a Sierra Club spokesperson: " 'When these animals arrive at the slaughterhouses, their hides are already filthy with manure from being raised in such confined spaces and they are more likely to be stressed, which helps create more pathogens.' Slaughter plants further exacerbate contamination problems as high-speed processing lines and the mixing of meat from many animals help spread bacteria."[19]

Pork, lamb, and some other animal products contain toxoplasma, which if acquired during pregnancy can lead to birth defects, miscarriage, and stillbirth. Any person with an immune system that is compromised can also have serious problems. And choosing fish over other kinds of animal food does not remove the danger of food poisoning. A recent *Consumer Reports* study found that more than 25% of the fish purchased from grocery stores by their shoppers were "on the brink of spoilage," and found unacceptable levels of methyl mercury and G. coli, a bacterium indicating the presence of fecal matter and possibly pathogens, in many of the samples.[20] Fish also contain incredible amounts of pesticides, PCBs, and other toxins, because they have to live in "civilization's sewer," the increasingly ruined waters of the planet. Fish farms contribute to the problem by breeding disease and parasites, putting abnormal stress on the animals and polluting ecologically fragile coastal waters.[21] And, since it takes five pounds of wild ocean fish to produce one pound of farmed saltwater fish or shrimp, "aquaculture" is also seen as a contributing factor to the depletion of fisheries worldwide.[22]

• ECOLOGICAL IMPLICATIONS

Even on land, raising animals for food is by far the greatest consumer and polluter of fresh water on the planet, draining off 60% of our continent's entire fresh water supply. A person eating a meat-based diet causes 6,000 gallons of water to be consumed every day, compared to the person on a plant-based diet, who uses about 300 gallons per day. In addition, huge amounts of toxic waste are generated by animals used for human food. The demand that omnivores and carnivores place on the environment is also responsible for the destruction of priceless and irreplaceable tropical rainforests in Africa, Central America, and South America, which help regulate Earth's temperature and air supply, and offer incredible promise in newfound plant-based medical research.[23] The Rainforest Action Network reported that 200,000,000 pounds of fresh and frozen beef was imported from Central American countries in 1993 and in 1994. Two thirds of these countries' rainforests have been cleared, primarily to raise cattle for export for U.S. food industry profit. The USDA Economic Research Service reports that the United States imports 78 million pounds of beef from Brazil every year, fed on destroyed rainforest converted to grazing land.[24] In their book *People of the Tropical Rainforest*, biologists Julie Denslow and Christine Padoch state that every fast-food hamburger made from rainforest beef represents a loss in life forms of twenty to thirty different plant species, 100 different insect species, and dozens of different bird, mammal, and reptile species.[25]

The American animal agricultural system is the most wasteful food production system in the world. The raising and processing of animals and animal products for human consumption requires 20 calories of energy for each one calorie of usable food energy returned. Only a fraction of the energy consumed by an animal or bird is left in the flesh and muscle at the time of slaughter. Therefore, the use of land to feed animals whose dead bodies will eventually feed humans is extremely wasteful and inefficient. Conversely, to grow plant crops, on average, we see that for every one calorie put into the soil, we reap 60 calories of usable food energy.

Scientific American magazine reported about twenty years ago that one pound of bacon requires ten times as much crop land as is needed to make one pound of soybean bacon analog. The vast majority of the grains and legumes grown in the U.S. are actually fed to animals. If Americans who eat animals decreased their animal flesh consumption by 10%, they would create a surplus of 12 million tons of grain annually, enough to completely eliminate starvation in both Africa and in the rest of America.

One of the main reasons for famine in many parts of the world is deforestation of land used to graze cattle. Further, trees shade the soil, and roots act as a pump to keep the water near the surface of the ground, helping to keep the water table high and the topsoil intact. With the trees cut down, the rainwater does not soak into the topsoil but runs off the hills and settles into valleys, taking precious topsoil with it. When soil is exposed to sun, wind, and rain, it is baked dry and either blows away or washes away into streams and rivers.

B. Jensen, M.D., and M. Anderson write in their book *Empty Harvest*: "No civilization has ever lived beyond the health of its soil, and only by artificial means have we stretched this rule and extended this civilization. Since modern farmers do not use soil-building techniques, it takes between 100 and 1,000 years for natural forces to form one inch of topsoil." Ninety percent of the 6 billion tons of topsoil eroded annually is American farmland. The United States Department of Agriculture estimates that a 6-inch loss of topsoil is capable of reducing crop yields by 40% per year. Good soil is 45% minerals, and one teaspoon of non-chemically treated soil hosts more living creatures than there are people in the world. The European settlers found 18 to 25 inches of rich topsoil in America in the sixteenth and seventeenth centuries; most farmlands today are working with a mere 6 to 9 inches of topsoil.[26] The Sanilac Conservation District's 48th Annual Report notes that total sheet and rill erosion on cropland in 1992 was 1.2 billion tons (or 3.1 tons per acre on 382 million acres). It states that controlling erosion "not only sustains the long-term productivity of the land, but also affects the amount of soil, pesticides, fertilizer, and other substances that move into the nation's waters."[27]

Unhealthy soil leads to unhealthy foods, an unhealthy environment, and, ultimately, unhealthy humans. Living, healthy, and abundant soil is transformed into lifeless and imbalanced soil by synthetic fertilizers, pesticides, and herbicides. Rather than striving to maintain the health of the soil and the plants that they grow, many farmers only invest in synthetic mineral supplements that will give their crops the mere appearance of health. Interestingly, Baron Justus von Liebig, the German chemist who discovered that nitrogen, phosphorous, and potassium were the main minerals necessary to force growth of plants that *resembled* healthy crops (this formula, called synthetic NPK, is now widely used by American commercial farmers), recanted his discovery in 1873 with deep remorse for his misguided contribution. Later, Julius Hensel wrote a book called *Bread from Stones*, revising the recommendation to farmers to utilize natural rock dust, which ultimately proved to produce strong and very high-quality, drought-resistant crops.[28] The presence of trace minerals, fungus, microbial life, etc. in the soil has been found to contribute immensely to the production of healthy crops.

An organic farmer will stick his or her hands into the soil, smell it, and test it for water retention, organic matter content, pH balance, mineral balance, and plant sugar content, understanding that sick plants will respond naturally to healthy soil. Organic farmers may use ladybugs, various worms, garlic juice, mulches, soaps, or other crops that repel insects naturally, rather than harmful and dangerous non-biodegradable chemicals. Rather than synthetic chemical fertilizer and hormones, an organic farmer will utilize seaweed, compost, organically fed animal manure, earthworms, fish meal, worm castings, bone meal, or lime. Nature knows just what to do with these natural substances. Synthetic chemicals, on the other hand, cause mass destruction, the likes of which we are only now beginning to understand.

Rachel Carson, the author of *Silent Spring*, one of the first books to draw widespread attention to the problem of toxins threatening the sustaining of life on our planet, quoted Dr. Albert Schweitzer: "Man has lost the capacity to foresee and to forestall. He will end by destroying the earth."[29] The amounts of oil, gas, and electricity we use in livestock farming, slaughter, and processing, and the extent of the irreversible harm we are doing to our air, water, and soil from pesticides, hormones, herbicides, antibiotics, genetic mutations, and animal waste is unfathomable. Our current methods are not working. (Those readers who are interested in the science and research that aimed to call attention to these matters decades ago may refer to the works of Sir Robert McCarrison, Rachel Carson, Dr. Francis Pottenger, Dr. Roger

Williams, Dr. Agnes Faye Morgan, Dr. Weston Price, Dr. Harvey Wiley, Dr. Royal Lee, Dr. William Albrecht, and Dr. Bernard Jensen.)

If we start to see Earth as a metaphor for our own bodies, we can also begin to observe the universal effect of short-sighted manipulation upon it. Earth's circulatory system is made of rivers, lakes, and oceans. Its skin is the fragile ozone layer. Both Earth and the human body are "closed systems," meaning that if you poison one area, the poison soon travels to another area. We are producing less nutritious food at the highest cost in history, while our farmers go bankrupt.[30] We saturate our bodies and the earth with chemicals to try to stop disease. Our culture is not simply "unnatural"; it has actually become "anti-natural." As we distance ourselves farther and faster from nature's cleansers, we are approaching a point of no return.

Buddha is quoted as saying, "As a net is made up by a series of ties, so everything in this world is connected by a series of ties. If anyone thinks that the mesh of a net is independent, isolated, then, he is mistaken."[31]

The Native Americans lived on this continent for several thousand years without disturbing the ecological balance or interfering with the land's ability to provide clothing, food, and other necessities for survival. A familiar quote from Chief Seattle states, "What befalls the earth befalls all the sons of the earth. . . . This we know: the earth does not belong to man, man belongs to earth. All things are connected like the blood that unites us all. Man did not weave the web of life, he is merely a strand in it. Whatever he does to the web, he does to himself."

Unfortunately, American settlers started the clearcutting of forests and depletion of soil. To date, over 260 million acres of American forests have been cleared for the production of animals for human food. The vast majority of the grain we grow goes to feed these animals, whom we raise in order to kill and consume. Begun in the 1800s, these practices have left North America with only 7 to 8 inches of topsoil left before we reach barren desert status.[32] As with other resource depletion problems, the U.S. simply exports short-sighted, unsustainable production practices to other countries.

Today, Americans need to demand more from ourselves and our government by refusing to intellectually and financially support any compromises to the truth about disease prevention and sustainable environmental balance. We need to put our own and the planet's health back in order before it is too late. In the pursuit of planetary health, all individuals and all nations become equal. We are all on the same team, and, if we act in accordance with what we know to be best for Earth and for ourselves, there will be life-sustaining work and healing for everyone.

1. McDougall, John A., M.D., *McDougall's Medicine: A Challenging Second Opinion* (Clinton, NJ: New Win Publishing, Inc., 1985), 289.
2. Barnard, Neal, M.D., *Food for Life* (New York: Three Rivers Press, 1993), 145.
3. Graff, Brian, "Health Experts Challenge 'New' Fat Recommendation," *Vegetarian Voice* Winter 1998; 22(4), 6–7, 26, 36 .
4. Tanner, J. M., "Trend towards earlier menarche in London, Oslo, Copenhagen, the Netherlands, and Hungary," *Nature* 1973; 243: 75–76.

5. Kagawa, Y., "Impact of Westernization on the nutrition of Japanese: changes in physique, cancer, longevity, and centenarians," *Preventive Medicine*, 1978; 7: 205–217.

6. Rose, D. P., Boyar, A. P., Cohen, C., and Strong, L. E., "Effect of a low-fat diet on hormone levels in women with cystic breast disease. 1. Serum steroids and gonadotropins," *Journal of the National Cancer Institute*, 1987; 78(4) 623–626.

    Ingram, D. M., Bennett, F. C., Willcox, D., and deKlerk, N., "Effect of a low-fat diet on female sex hormone levels," *Journal of the National Cancer Institute*, 1987; 79(6): 1225–1229.

    Goldin, B.R., Adlercreutz, H., Gorbach, S. L., et al., "Estrogen excretion patterns and plasma levels in vegetarian and omnivorous women," *New England Journal of Medicine*, 1982; 307: 1542–1547.

    Barnard, *Food for Life*, 25–28.

7. de Ridder, C. M., Thijssen, J. H. H., Van't Veer, P., et al., "Dietary habits, sexual maturation, and plasma hormones in pubertal girls: a longitudinal study," *American Journal of Clinical Nutrition*, 1991; 54: 805–813.

8. Barnard, *Food for Life*, 28.

9. "European Union Says Beef Hormone Can Cause Cancer," *Meat Industry Insights*, May 3, 1999, cited in Robbins, John, *The Food Revolution* (Berkeley, CA: Conari Press, 2001), 143.

10. Ibid., 142.

11. Clyde D. Lane Jr., Professor, Extension Animal Science (Beef, Sheep, Horses), University of Tennessee, www.mycattle.com (adapted from "Guide to Assuring Beef Quality on the Farm," written by the Kentucky Beef Cattle Association, 1992).

12. Keeler, Barbara, and Marc Lappé, "Some Food for FDA Regulation," *Los Angeles Times*, January 7, 2001, cited in Robbins, *Food Revolution*, 336.

13. Robbins, *Food Revolution*, 336–337.

14. Hergenrather, J., et al., "Pollutants in Breast Milk of Vegetarians," a letter in the *New England Journal of Medicine* 1976; 304: 792.

15. Jensen, Bernard, M.D., and Mark Anderson, *Empty Harvest: Understanding the Link between Our Food, Our Immunity, and Our Planet* (New York: Avery Publishing, 1990), 69.

16. *Consumer Reports*, Fall 1997, cited in *Veggie Life* magazine, July 1998, 14.

17. Barnard, *Food for Life*, 134–135.

18. Robbins, *Food Revolution*, 192–196.

19. Farmed Animal Watch, Oct. 16, 2002, Issue #89; http://www.farmedanimal.net/Newsletters/Newsletter89.htm.

20. "America's Fish: Fair or Foul?" *Consumer Reports*, February 2001.

21. People for the Ethical Treatment of Animals, 2002.

22. Robbins, *Food Revolution*, 298.

23. Robbins, John, *Diet For a New America* video (California: KCET Video, Community Television of Southern California, 1991), cited in Klaper, Michael, M.D., *Pregnancy, Children, and the Vegan Diet* (Kapa'au, Hawaii: Gentle World, Inc., 1994), 70–71.

24. Barnard, *Food for Life*, xvii.

25. Robbins, *Food Revolution*, 256–257.

26. Jensen and Anderson, *Empty Harvest*, 4–5; 31–33.

27. "Sanilac County Conservation District's 48th Annual Report," *Sanilac County News*, July 1998.

28. von Liebig, Justus, *Agricultural Chemistry* (1855) and *The Natural Laws of Husbandry* (1870), and Hensel, Julius, *Bread from Stones*, cited in Jensen and Anderson, *Empty Harvest*, 74–75.

29. Carson, Rachel L., *Silent Spring* (Connecticut: Crest Books, 1962), cited in Jensen and Anderson, *Empty Harvest*, xi.

30. Jensen and Anderson, *Empty Harvest*, 14.

31. Ibid., 26.

32. Ibid., foreword.

9

CONCLUSION

DIETARY CONSIDERATIONS IN THE PREVENTION and treatment of chronic disease have previously been thrown into the category of "alternative medicine," along with techniques such as acupressure, energy medicine, and homeopathy—the assumption being that these techniques were inferior to the real business of "conventional medicine." However, the current trend toward "integrative medicine" shows acknowledgment that there are times when one approach may be better than the other, or times when both approaches are necessary. For example, an acute, bleeding car accident victim requires conventional diagnosis, treatment, and possibly surgery, but the role of proper diet in the healing process will also be acknowledged. In chronic disease prevention situations, however, the most effective approach has been prudent management of controllable lifestyle factors, such as exercise, stress, diet, and asbestos, pesticides, tobacco smoke, and other pollutants. I believe that there will come a day when it constitutes malpractice for doctors not to inform their patients of all of their options, including lifestyle and dietary changes that can reverse and prevent the diseases mentioned throughout this book. Perhaps before long we will take our cue from Europe, where some insurance premiums are lowered for vegtetarians, as is customarily done for nonsmokers and drivers with safe records.

One of the problems in educating our citizens about dietary prevention of chronic disease is a general belief that vegetarians live on lettuce and go hungry all the time. As noted earlier in detail, a person on a vegan diet could eat almost twice as much as in volume—with no ill health effects—as someone eating the SAD of meat, dairy, fats, oils, and sweets. For example, you'll find the same number of calories in 1 1/2 whole cups of fresh, cool watermelon as you would in about three bites of one unfrosted Pop-Tart! The watermelon satisfies the appetite without putting the consumer at risk for the chronic diseases discussed earlier in this book. And, by not overloading the body with fat and toxins, the vegan diet allows us to function more efficiently. As we consider a few of the tasks the human body performs each day, it becomes clear that proper maintenance is essential for optimal health.

The average adult consumes between 1 and 5 pounds of food, and utilizes 2.75 quarts of water, per day.[1] Humans have 100 trillion cells, 600 muscles, and 206 bones. The average human adult can listen to information at the rate of 300 words per minute and speak at the rate of 200 words per minute. Our bodies manufacture up to 5,000,000 cells per second (each cell lasts about four months before being replaced), and our blood is carried through our bodies via 70,000 miles of circulatory blood vessels (which equals about 15 feet underneath each square inch of skin).[2] These functions, and thousands more, are carried out without our conscious knowledge, until the average American dies at the age of 77 years.[3] If we begin to see the human body as an intricate, miraculous machine—capable of such astounding feats as metabolic and chemical synthesis and cell regeneration—we come to respect it, and begin to take care what we put into it. The New Testament of the Bible states in I Timothy 2:5, "The body is the Temple of the Lord." Indeed, and what a charge we are given to care for it!

It's not too late to begin taking good care of your body, no matter how long you've lived by the Basic Four Food Groups, the Food Pyramid, or the menu of your local fast food chain. In fact, it is interesting to observe that the body, fed properly, loses its "taste" for junk food in a relatively short period of time, regardless of how many years one has followed the SAD. Research on over 2,000 women at the University of Washington in Seattle showed that after limiting fat intake for up to six months, the participants reported that fatty foods were actually unpleasant to eat. Dr. Dean Ornish's studies are revealing the same effects in his patients on a lowered-fat diet. He further states that there was a direct correlation between the amount of change his patients made and the extent to which they improved.[4] And Dr. Kenneth Greenspan, working at the Columbia Presbyterian Hospital's Laboratory and Center for Stress Related Disorders in New York, noted "tremendous enthusiasm and adherence" to the macrobiotic and natural foods diet used to control angina pectoris, blood pressure, and other coronary risk factors.[5]

These findings fly in the face of the American government officials' statements that they don't want to make dietary suggestions that might be just "too difficult" for Americans to follow. Dr. McDougall, who has said that the quarter-million coronary artery bypass operations that take place annually in the U.S. are ineffective in the long run, states, "Few individuals will risk being sick again when they know how to avoid such episodes of stress."[6] Consumers will also find the vegan diet attractive in financial terms, since it was found by one source to reduce grocery bills by about 40%.[7] According to a George Washington University study, the diet offers a savings of $2,100 annually for the average family of four.[8]

Thankfully, trends in industrialized countries are beginning to show evidence of a change from high-fat, high-cholesterol, animal-based diets. For example, the number of vegetarians in Great Britain doubled between 1983 and 1994.[9]

At a recent presentation about vegetarian nutrition and the implementation of foods to meet nutritional requirements at the National Association of College and University Food Services Region II Conference in Pennsylvania, Debra Wasserman asked the audience of about forty-five represented universities how many attendees had vegans eating in their dining halls. Every single attendee raised a hand.[10] Awareness and demand are growing at a grassroots level.

Another survey, this one done by the *Vegetarian Journal* in 1997 on 717 respondents, broke down the stated reasons for interest in a vegetarian diet, and noted the respondents' education level compared to the general population, among other measures. Eighty-two percent said they were interested in vegetarianism because of health issues, 75% because of ethical issues such as animal rights and the environment, 31% because of taste, and 26% because of economic reasons (apparently, respondents were allowed to choose more than one reason). The survey respondents were highly educated when compared to the general population. Ninety-one percent had attended college for some period of time. A breakdown showed that 35% had completed one college degree, 27% held a master's degree, and 5% held doctorates in medicine or philosophy.[11]

Americans seem to be upgrading their expectations for quality in agriculture. A November 1988 Harris Poll checked public opinion about organic food production vs. commercially grown food. Over 84% of those polled said that they would rather buy organically grown food than commercially grown food with pesticides and fertilizers added, and 49% said that they would be willing to pay more money for this organic food.[12] It is estimated that these figures are even higher today.

In 1998, the author sent a letter to Michigan's U.S. Senator Carl Levin, urging a vote to oppose the USDA's attempts at pushing through legislation that would allow their standards on "organic agricultural products" to include the use of antibiotics, irradiation, biotechnology, genetic engineering, and the use of sewage sludge fertilizer. In a response letter dated May 27, 1998, Senator Levin noted that the Secretary of Agriculture had rejected the current proposal and was calling for major revisions in the proposed legislation "as a result of the 200,000 comments" received from taxpayers. This public outcry pushed the USDA to revise their definition of "organic," and today the USDA organic seal can only be displayed on products that are 95–100% organic. Dan Glickman, the Agricultural Secretary stated, "If organic farmers and consumers reject our national standards, we have failed."[13]

As a result of citizen uprisings all over the world, many corporations and governments have initiated labeling standards or bans on all GMO products. After the Aventis Starlink corn disaster, in which 9 million bushels of corn deemed unfit for human consumption ended up in 300 different types of foods, Americans were outraged. By late 2000, the term "frankenfood" was becoming a buzzword, and 33% of Americans said that farmers should no longer be allowed to grow genetically altered crops.[14]

Other positive changes include the American Dietetic Association's update to their 1993 position paper on vegetarian diets, which originally stated meekly that "vegetarian diets are healthful and nutritionally adequate when appropriately planned." The revision notes that vegetarian diets are higher in folate, antioxidants, and phytochemicals, all of which have disease-protective effects. Their new statement reads, "It is the position of the American Dietetic Association that vegetarian diets are nutritionally adequate and provide health benefits in the prevention and treatment of certain diseases."

The update also contained a new vegetarian food guide pyramid for meal planning, along with two items that put to rest certain concerns about vegetarianism that conventional medicine has habitually professed. First, it states that "protein combining" is not necessary, and that protein intake in vegetarians and vegans appears to be adequate. Incidentally, Dr. John McDougall is taking this concept one step further, by directly challenging health organizations that continue to claim that complete amino acids are only found in animals and animal by-products. Secondly, the ADA update states that vegans may have lower calcium requirements than the general population, because their diets contain less protein and more alkaline foods, whereas high-acid diets cause more calcium to be lost in the urine as the body tries to neutralize the acidity caused during the digestion of animal flesh and fluids, with calcium from the bones.[15] The update was prompted by the Vegetarian Nutrition Dietetic Practice group of the ADA, who felt the original position needed to be updated to reflect the vast amount of scientific data verifying the health advantages of a vegetarian way of life.

Another positive sign is the new nationally approved "Meals on Wheels" vegan menu plan option for senior citizens. One thousand locations in the United States have already received information packets on this new option through Vegetarian Resource Group supporters.[16]

While many of today's restaurants have menus that are animal-flesh-centered, one can usually find something on the menu that does not contain fat or cholesterol. Sometimes, however, it is nearly impossible, as even the well-intentioned restaurateur who includes a "heart-healthy pasta" will typically use a cream sauce, or pile cow-milk cheese on top of the tomato sauce covering a bleached and chemically enriched noodle product. If you are dining out and see grease and oil on the plate or on the packaging, remember that this is what you have just chosen to put into your precious body! But there are signs that things will be changing soon, as noted in a recent article regarding 75 restaurant chains and their intentions to be "vegetarian- and vegan-friendly."[17] Further,

Technomics, a consultant to the food service industry, cited the demand for meatless products as one of the fastest-growing consumer trends.[18]

Even the National Aeronautics and Space Administration (NASA), as it proceeds with plans for missions to Mars, and other missions lasting more than three years, has embraced plant-based meals as the most efficient way to obtain nourishment in space, just as it is on Earth. NASA has acknowledged the superior sustainability of a plant-based diet over an animal-based diet in its miniature model ecosystems, and is working with researchers at Cornell University to implement a sustainable, plant-based diet including wheat, sweet potatoes, rice, beans, peppers, tomatoes, carrots, lettuce and herbs, grown hydroponically.[19] Limited by space and weight constraints, we can see the analogy between the closed system of a spacecraft and the closed system of our planet, and its implications.

Eating for optimal health becomes simpler when we look at the natural environment of foods and our human capabilities. When observing cautions regarding plant fats, for example, you could imagine yourself in the midst of plant foods in their natural habitat. The digging, climbing, shelling, hulling, and so forth that would be necessary to obtain nuts, seeds, and coconuts are time-consuming, and indicate that their consumption would naturally be in smaller amounts than other plants, such as apples, grapes, or corn, which are easily picked or gathered, and can be eaten with little or no preparation.

Whole food health advocates say to eat plant foods that are as raw, fresh, whole, and organic as possible. For those who choose to cook, the following food preparation rules are simple and easy to follow.

If you choose to boil food, use as little water as possible, use a lid, and boil the food for as short a time as possible. These simple measures can help preserve precious vitamins, minerals, and other phytonutrients. Cooking food can alter fiber quality, leading many experts to recommend a general increase in the amount of raw foods in the human diet.

Cooking with animal-derived fats introduces unnecessary and harmful cholesterol, fat, and calories into your body, yet it has become common in the SAD to add grease, butter, or oil to almost everything eaten. As you clean the dishes and pans when dining at home, picture those substances you are scrubbing away, now inside your body. If you are still eating animals and animal products, and therefore are scrubbing pans with metal scrapers, steel wool, scrub solutions, and chemical detergents, ask yourself if this is what you want in your arteries, and in the cells of your living body! Further, ask yourself how long it will take—and at what cost—for your body to identify, metabolize, and eliminate this grease, as well as the hormones, antibiotics, bacteria, etc. that you have taken into your body, from your organs, bloodstream, fat stores, muscles, etc. This is a helpful reminder at every meal. Removing the grease from your diet will make weight regulation so much simpler, and your body will be able to perform all of its functions (including metabolism and regulation) so much more efficiently when its energy is not wasted on trying to eliminate disease-promoting toxins. Many disease processes have been proven to be reversed by the elimination of fats and oils, notably ath-

erosclerosis, angina, hormone imbalances, adult-type diabetes, inflammatory arthritis, attacks of multiple sclerosis,
acne, oily skin, and gallbladder disease.[20]

When selecting pre-packaged foods, be aware of what
the labeling really means. Be aware, too, that manufacturers
will manipulate statistics in their ads—for example, a product that is "91% fat-free" by weight may still have a high
percentage of calories from fat. *Calorie-free* means up to 5
calories per serving, *low-calorie* means 40 or fewer calories
per serving, and *sugar-free* means up to .5 grams of sugar per
serving (sugar-free foods often contain aspartame or saccharin, artificial sweeteners that come with their own set of
warnings). *Fat-free* means up to .5 grams of fat per serving.
Low-fat means up to 3 grams of fat per serving, or per 100
grams of the item. *Lite/Light* products contain one-third
fewer calories than the usual or original product *or* 50% less
fat than the same serving size of the regular product.[21] The fat
in these foods has often been replaced with potentially dangerous chemical substitutes. Some of these additives are touted as inert or indigestible, or could be reasonably labeled as
harmful, yet the products remain available for sale. The
author recommends using extreme caution with products
containing the fat substitute Olestra, due to complaints by
consumers and the commonsense question: If it is true that
we are ingesting a substance that is "not digestible" by
humans, what happens when a little bit leaks out through the
intestines and enters the bloodstream through an ulcer,
wound, esophageal varices, etc.? Some evidence suggests that
Olestra may cause cancer and liver problems.[22]

Making only a slight change in your diet, like switching from ice cream to frozen yogurt or from beef to chicken, gives you the worst of both worlds—a sense of deprivation without feeling better, looking better, or functioning better. However, we can have the best of both worlds—a healthy life through a healthy diet, founded in a deeper understanding of the wisdom of nature's own balances.

It is a simple truth that for our own survival we need to learn to work with nature rather than try to somehow fool its cycles or conquer its forces—for nature is within us, quite literally. We cannot control or escape it; it is the fabric of everything around us. It is not something "out there" that must be "tamed," but something "in here"—in our own bodies. The food choices described in this book are founded in an awareness of the interconnectedness of humans and the environment, for "studying ecological and social systems in isolation of one another is no longer tenable."[23]

Upon completing the research and literature for this book, I came to the conclusion that ecosystem interconnectedness should be taught in every family, in every school, and in every business. The awareness that every decision we make affects the life of the planet as a whole, and thereby our own survival, should be the foundation of the community mindset in its decisions to change the status quo. Decisions made at any level would have to pass a commonsense test based on the ecosystem model: is a given practice sustainable in a small biosphere over the long term? How about, for example, factory farming? Deforestation? Is being violent or tyrannical to other living things good for the ecosystem? How about polluting the air we all breathe?

If we know that a plant-based diet is superior for human health, helps to prevent animal abuse, helps to preserve topsoil, rainforests, air and water quality, and feeds more humans than an animal-based diet, what are we waiting for? What are you waiting for?

1. McDougall, John A., M.D., *McDougall's Medicine: A Challenging Second Opinion* (Clinton, NJ: New Win Publishing, Inc., 1985), 64.
2. Wagman, Richard, M.D., F.A.C.P., ed. *The New Complete Medical and Health Encyclopedia, Vol. 1* (Chicago: J. G. Ferguson Publishing Company: 1987), 2–45.
3. Pawlak, Laura, Ph.D., R.D., lecture on *Alternative Medicine: An Objective View* (Emeryville, CA: Institute for Natural Resources, 1998), Troy, Michigan, June 1998.
4. Barnard, Neal, M.D., *Food for Life* (New York: Three Rivers Press, 1993), 53.
   Bricklin, Mark, ed. *Your Perfect Weight* (Prevention: Rodale Press, Inc., 1995), 26.
5. Kushi, Michio, and Jack, Alex, *Diet for a Strong Heart* (New York: St. Martin's Press, 1985), 131.
6. McDougall, John A., M.D., *The McDougall Program* (New York: Penguin Group, 1990), 12–13.
7. Ibid., 11.
8. Barnard, *Food for Life*, xii.
9. Johnston, Patricia K., Dr.P.H., M.S., R.D., *Loma Linda University Vegetarian Nutrition & Health Newsletter* 1997, Vol. 1, No. 1, 4.
10. Vogel, Michael, "Notes From the Scientific Department: Outreach," *Vegetarian Journal*, January–February 1998, Vol. 17, No. 1, 18.
11. Wasserman, Debra, and Charles Stahler, cited in *Vegetarian Journal*, January–February 1998, Vol. 17, No. 1, 4.
12. Harris, Louis and Associates (Poll shows that public prefers organic food), *Organic Gardening*, November, 1988, cited in Jensen, Bernard, M.D., and Mark Anderson, *Empty Harvest: Understanding the Link between Our Food, Our Immunity, and Our Planet* (New York: Avery Publishing, 1990), 66.

13. McIntee, Gerard, "Nutritional News," *Energy Times*, July–August 1998, 12.

14. Robbins, John, *The Food Revolution* (Berkeley, CA: Conari Press, 2001), 379.

15. Messina, Virginia, M.P.H., R.D., and Kenneth Burke, Ph.D., R.D., "American Dietetic Association Position Paper on Vegetarian Diets," *Journal of the American Dietetic Association* 1997; 97: 1317–1321.

16. Vogel, Michael, "Meals on Wheels and the VRG Collaborate to Bring Vegetarian Meals to Nation's Seniors," and "Position of the American Dietetic Association on Vegetarian Diets is Updated," *Vegetarian Journal*, January–February 1998, Vol. 17, No. 1, back cover.

17. Bartas, Jeanne-Marie, "Vegan Menu Items at Fast Food and Family-Style Restaurants—Part II," in *Vegetarian Journal*, January–February 1998, Vol. 17, No. 1, 24.

18. Johnston, *Loma Linda University Vegetarian Nutrition and Health Newsletter*, 4.

19. http://health.discovery.com.

20. McDougall, John A., M.D., and Mary McDougall, *The New McDougall Cookbook* (New York: Penguin Group, 1993), 14.

21. Bricklin, *Your Perfect Weight*, 44, 352–353.

22. Barnard, *Food for Life*, 107.

23. Low, B., et al. 1999. "Human Ecosystem Interactions: A Dynamic Integrated Model." *Ecological Economics* (20), 227–42.

BIBLIOGRAPHY

✠

The American Heart Association Heartbook, New York: Dutton, 1980.

"A multiple share of myeloma," *Medical World News,* May 16, 1969; 23.

Anonymous, "Contribution of the microflora of the small intestine to the vitamin B12 nutriture of man," *Nutrition Reviews* August 1980; 38(8): 274.

Appleby, P., et al., "The Oxford Vegetarian Study: An Overview," *American Journal of Clinical Nutrition* 1999; 70(3): 525S–531S.

Armstrong, B., "Urinary sodium and blood pressure in vegetarians," *American Journal of Clinical Nutrition* 1979; 32: 2472.

Astrand, Per-Olf, "Something Old and Something New . . . Very New," *Nutrition Today* 1968; 3(2): 9–11.

Barnard, Neal, M.D., *Food for Life,* New York: Three Rivers Press, 1993.

Berenson, G. S., et al., "Cardiovascular Risk Factors in Children and Early Prevention of Heart Disease," *Clinical Chemistry* 1988; 34: B115–122.

Bethwaite, P., et al., "Adult-onset acute leukemia in employment in the meat industry: a New Zealand case-control study," *Cancer Causes and Control* 2001; 12: 635–643.

Blankenhorn, D. H., et al., "Beneficial effects of combined colestipol-niacin therapy on coronary atherosclerosis and coronary venous bypass grafts," *Journal of the American Medical Association* 1987; 257: 3233–3240.

Bricklin, Mark, ed. *Your Perfect Weight*, Prevention: Rodale Press, Inc., 1995.

Brody, Jane E., "Research Yields Surprises About Early Human Diets," *New York Times*, Science Section, May 15, 1979.

Burkitt, D., "Varicose Veins, Deep Vein Thrombosis and Hemorrhoids: Epidemiology and Suggested Aetiology," *British Medical Journal* 1972; 2: 556.

——., and James, P., "Low-Residue Diets and Hiatus Hernia," *Lancet* 1973; 2: 128–130.

Burr, M., "Plasma cholesterol and blood pressure in vegetarians," *Journal of Human Nutrition* 1981; 35: 437.

"The Case Against Heated Milk Protein," *Atherosclerosis* 1971; January–February, 13: 137–139.

Castelli, W. P., "Epidemiology of coronary heart disease," *American Journal of Medicine* 1984; 76 (2A): 4–12.

——., "Summary of Lessons from the Framingham Heart Study," Framingham, Massachusetts, September 1983.

Connor, W., "The key role of nutritional factors in the prevention of coronary artery disease," *Preventive Medicine* 1972; 1: 49.

Cramer, D., et al., "Galactose Consumption and Metabolism in Relation to the Risk of Ovarian Cancer," *Lancet* 1989; 2: 66–71.

Davis, Brenda, and Vesanto Melina, *Becoming Vegan*, Summertown, TN: Book Publishing Company, 2000.

De Ridder, C. M., Thijssen, J. H. H., Van't Veer, P., et al., "Dietary habits, sexual maturation, and plasma hormones in pubertal girls: a longitudinal study," *American Journal of Clinical Nutrition*, 1991; 54: 805–813.

Draper, H., "Calcium, phosphorous, and osteoporosis," *Fed. Proc.* 1981; 40: 2434.

Drogan, J., et. al. "Fatty diet affects girls' hormones: Cutting fat may slow puberty, lower breast cancer risk," cited by Reuters, January 15, 2003, at www.msnbc.com/news/859863.asp?0si=-&cp1=1.

Eaton, S. B., and Konner, M., "Paleolithic Nutrition," *New England Journal of Medicine* 1995; 313: 283–289.

Editorial: "Diet and ischemic heart disease: agreement or not?" *Lancet* 1983; 2: 317.

Edmonds, Brian, *The Doctors' Book of Bible Healing Foods*, Boca Raton, FL: Globe Communications Corp., 1992.

Elliott, S. S., et al., "Fructose, weight gain, and the insulin resistance syndrome," *American Journal of Clinical Nutrition* 2002; 76(5): 911–922.

Ellis, F., et al., "Incidence of Osteoporosis in Vegetarians and Omnivores," *American Journal of Clinical Nutrition* 1974; 27: 916.

———., "Veganism, Clinical Findings and Investigations," *American Journal of Clinical Nutrition*, March 1976; Vol. 23, No. 3, 249–255.

Energy Times magazine, July–August 1998.

Englyst, H. N., et al., "Nonstarch Polysaccharide Concentrations in Four Scandinavian Populations," *Nutrition & Cancer* 1982; 4: 50–60.

Enos, W., "Pathogenesis of coronary artery disease in American soldiers killed in Korea," *Journal of the American Medical Association* 1955; 158: 912.

Esselstyn, C. B., "Resolving the Coronary Artery Disease Epidemic through Plant-Based Nutrition," *Preventive Cardiology* 2001; 4: 171–177.

Farmed Animal Watch, October 16, 2002, Issue 89, www.farmedanimal.net/Newsletters/Newsletter89.htm.

Ferrer, J. "Milk of dairy cows frequently contains a leukemogenic virus," *Science* 1981; 213: 1014–1015.

Fisher, I., "The Influence of Flesh Eating on Endurance," *Yale Medical Journal* 1907; 13: 205–221.

Food Balance Sheets, 1979–1981, Average, Rome: FAO, 1984.

"Further Evidence in the Case Against Heated Milk Protein," *Atherosclerosis* 1972; January–February, 15: 129.

Goldin, B. R., et al., "Estrogen excretion patterns and plasma levels in vegetarian and omnivorous women," *New England Journal of Medicine* 1982; 307(25): 1542–1547.

Gregorio, D. I., Emrich, L. J., Graham, S., Marshall, J. R., and Nemoto, T., "Dietary fat consumption and survival among women with breast cancer," *Journal of the National Cancer Institute* 1985; 254: 2728.

Grimes, D., "Refined Carbohydrate, Smooth-Muscle Spasm and Disease of the Colon," *Lancet* 1976; 1: 395–397.

Hartroft, W., "The incidence of coronary artery disease in patients treated with Sippy diet," *American Journal of Clinical Nutrition* 1964; 15: 205.

Heaney, R. "Calcium nutrition and bone health in the elderly American," *Journal of Clinical Nutrition* 1982; 36: 986.

Hegsted, M. "Urinary calcium and calcium balance in young men as affected by level of protein and phosphorous intake," *Journal of Nutrition* 1981; 111: 553.

Hergenrather, J., et al., "Pollutants in Breast Milk of Vegetarians," a letter in the *New England Journal of Medicine* 1976; 304: 792.

Hesler, J. R., et al., "LDL-induced cytotoxicity and its inhibition by HDL in human vascular smooth muscle and endothelial cells in culture," *Atherosclerosis* 1979; 32: 213.

Holman, R., "The natural history of atherosclerosis. The early aortic lesions as seen in New Orleans in the middle of the 20th century," *American Journal of Pathology* 1958; 34: 209.

Hosford, C., ed., "Medical Updates—Monounsaturated Fats Cut Breast Cancer Risk," in *Life Extension* magazine, Vol. 4, No. 7, 24.

Ingram, D. M., et al., "Effect of a low-fat diet on female sex hormone levels," *Journal of the National Cancer Institute*, 1987; 79(6): 1225–1229.

Inter Press Service/*TerraViva*, February 9, 2001.

Jack, Alex, *Let Food Be Thy Medicine,* Becket, MA: One Peaceful World Press, 1991.

Jensen, Bernard, M.D., and Mark Anderson, *Empty Harvest: Understanding the Link between Our Food, Our Immunity, and Our Planet,* New York: Avery Publishing, 1990.

Johnston, Patricia K., Dr.P.H., M.S., R.D., *Loma Linda University Vegetarian Nutrition & Health Newsletter 1997*, Vol. 1, No. 1.

Kagawa, Y., "Impact of Westernization on the nutrition of Japanese: changes in physique, cancer, longevity, and centenarians," *Preventive Medicine* 1978; 7: 205–217.

Katz, David, et. al., "Diet in the Prevention and Control of Obesity, Insulin Resistance, and Type II Diabetes: American College of Preventive Medicine Position Statement," American College of Preventive Medicine, 2002.

Klaper, Michael, M.D., *Pregnancy, Children, and the Vegan Diet,* Kapa'au, Hawaii: Gentle World, Inc., 1994.

Knuiman, J. T., and West, C. E., "The Concentration of Cholesterol in Serum and in Various Serum Lipoproteins in Macrobiotic, Vegetarian, and Non-vegetarian Men and Boys," *Atherosclerosis* 1983; 43: 71–82.

Koop, C. Everett, and the United States Department of Health and Human Services, Public Health Service, *The Surgeon General's Report on Nutrition and Health,* California: Prima Publishing, 1988, and New York: St. Martin's Press, 1988.

Korenblat, P., "Immune responses of human adults after oral and parenteral exposure to bovine serum albumin," *Journal of Allergy* 1968; 41: 226.

Kushi, L. H., et al., "Diet and 20-year Mortality from Coronary Heart Disease. The Ireland-Boston Diet-Heart Study," *New England Journal of Medicine* 1985; 312: 811–818.

Kushi, Michio, and Jack, Alex, *Diet for a Strong Heart,* New York: St. Martin's Press, 1985.

Lindahl, O., et al., "Vegan Diet Regimen with Reduced Medication in the Treatment of Bronchial Asthma," *Journal of Asthma* 1985; 22: 45–55.

Linkswiler, H., "Calcium retention of young adult males as affected by level of protein and calcium intake," *New York Academy of Science* 1974; 36: 333.

Low, B., et al., "Human Ecosystem Interactions: A Dynamic Integrated Model," *Ecological Economics* 1999; 20:227–42.

Lucas, P., "Dietary fat aggravates active rheumatoid arthritis," *Clinical Research* 1981; 29: 754A.

Mazess, R., "Bone mineral content of North Alaskan Eskimos," *American Journal of Clinical Nutrition* 1974; 27: 916–925.

McDougall, John A., M.D., *McDougall's Medicine: A Challenging Second Opinion,* Clinton, NJ: New Win Publishing, Inc., 1985.

———., *The McDougall Program,* New York: Penguin Group, 1990.

———., and Mary McDougall, *The New McDougall Cookbook,* New York: Penguin Group, 1993.

McIntyre, Gail F., M.D., J.D., "Alternatives to Hormone Replacement Therapy for Perimenopausal and Menopausal Symptoms" (presentation preparation overview), March 13, 2003, Mercy Health Center, Port Huron, MI.

Mead Johnson Nutritionals, *Enfamil Family of Formulas: Expressing & Storing Breastmilk,* Indiana: Mead Johnson & Co., 1996, 1997.

Messina, Virginia, M.P.H., R.D., and Burke, Kenneth, Ph.D., R.D., "American Dietetic Association Position Paper on Vegetarian Diets," *Journal of the American Dietetic Association* 1997; 97: 1317–1321.

"Milk Protein and Other Food Antigens in Atheroma and Coronary Heart Disease," *American Heart Journal* February 1971; 81: 189.

"A Multiple Share of Myeloma," *Medical World News,* May 16, 1969; 23.

National Osteoporosis Foundation: *Executive Summary of Osteoporosis.* Washington, D.C.: Osteoporosis International, 1998.

Neergard, Laura, "Many Women Quit Hormones," Associated Press, Thursday, October 24, 2002.

N.I.H. Consensus Development Conference Statement: "Lowering blood cholesterol to prevent heart disease," *Journal of the American Medical Association* 1985; 253: 2080.

Nixon, Daniel M., M.D., and Alison Brown, *The Cancer Recovery Eating Plan,* New York: Cerier Book Development, Inc., 1994/1996.

Norris, Jack, R.D. "Vegetarian and Vegan Diets: Health Implications," www.veganoutreach.org/health.

"Nutrition Recommendations for Canadians," *Canadian Medical Association Journal* 1971; 120 (10): 1241–1242.

Ophir, O., "Low blood pressure in vegetarians: the possible role of potassium," *American Journal of Clinical Nutrition* 1983; 37: 755.

Ornish, Dean, M.D., et al., "Can Lifestyle Changes Reverse Coronary Heart Disease?" *Lancet* 1990; 336: 129–133.

Oski, F., *Don't Drink Your Milk!*, New York: Mollica Press, Ltd., 1983.

——., "Is bovine milk a health hazard?" *Pediatrics* 1985; 75 (Supplement): 182.

Page, Lot B., M.D., "Epidemiologic Evidence on the Etiology of Human Hypertension and Its Possible Prevention," *American Heart Journal* 1976; 91: 527–534.

Parke, A. L. "Rheumatoid Arthritis and Food: A Case Study," *British Medical Journal* (Clinical research) June 20, 1981; 282 (6281): 2027–2029.

Pawlak, Laura, Ph.D., R.D., *Alternative Medicine: An Objective View: Biomed Seminar Course Pack*, 3rd. ed., Emeryville, CA: Institute for Natural Resources, 1998.

——., lecture on *Alternative Medicine: An Objective View* (Emeryville, CA: Institute for Natural Resources, 1998), Troy, Michigan, June 1998.

——., *A Perfect 10: Phyto "New-trients" against Cancers,* California: Biomed General Corporation, 1998.

——., *Weight Matters*, Emeryville, CA: Institute for Natural Resources/Biomed, 1998.

Pitchford, Paul, *Healing With Whole Foods, Revised,* California: North Atlantic Books, 1993.

Pritikin, Nathan, and Patrick McGrady, *The Pritikin Program for Diet and Exercise,* New York: Grosset and Dunlap, Inc., 1979.

Reaven, Gerald. "Dr. Gerald Reaven and Syndrome X," an interview by Robert Crayhon, M.S., at www.dfhi.com.

Robbins, J., *Diet For a New America* video, California: KCET Video, Community Television of Southern California, 1991.

——., *The Food Revolution*, Berkeley, CA: Conari Press, 2001.

Robertson, T. L., et al., "Epidemiologic Studies of Coronary Heart Disease and Stroke in Japanese Men Living in Japan, Hawaii, and California," *American Journal of Cardiology* 1977; 39: 239–243.

Rogers, Paul G., "Ensuring a Healthier Future," *Life Extension* magazine 1998, Vol. 4, No. 7, 19.

Rose, D. P., et al., "Effect of a low-fat diet on hormone levels in women with cystic breast disease. 1. Serum steroids and gonadotropins," *Journal of the National Cancer Institute*, 1987; 78(4) 623–626.

Sacks, F. M., Rosner, Bernard, and Kass, Edward H., "Blood Pressure in Vegetarians," *American Journal of Epidemiology* 1974; 100: 390–398.

Salonen, J. T., Salonen, R., Nyyssonen, K., and Korpela, H., "Iron sufficiency is associated with hypertension and excess risk of myocardial infarction: the Kuopio Ischaemic Heart Disease Risk Factor Study (KIHD)," *Circulation* 1992; 85: 864.

Sanilac County Conservation District's 48th Annual Report, *Sanilac County News*, Croswell, MI: Sanilac County News, July 1998.

Shekelle, R. B., et al., "Dietary Vitamin A and Risk of Cancer in the Western Electric Study," *Lancet* 1981; 2: 1185–1190.

Simone, Charles B., M.D. *Cancer and Nutrition*, New York: Avery Publishing Group, Inc., 1992.

Skoldstam, L, "Fasting and Vegan Diet in Rheumatoid Arthritis," *Scandinavian Journal of Rheumatology* 1987; 15 (2): 219–221.

Smith, R. W., Jr., and J. Rizek, "Epidemiologic studies of osteoporosis in women of Puerto Rico and Southeastern Michigan with special reference to age, race, national origin and to other related or associated findings. *Clinical Orthopaedics and Related Research* 1966; 45: 31–48.

Solomon, L. "Osteoporosis and fracture of the femoral neck in the South African Bantu," *Journal of Bone Joint Surgery* 1968; 50B: 2.

Stamler, J., "Lifestyles, major risk factors, proof, and public policy," *Circulation* 1978; 58: 3.

Stunkard, A. J., M.D., *Obesity and the social environment: Current status, future prospects*, in G. A. Bray, ed.: *Obesity in America*, N.I.H. Publication #80-359, 1980.

Tanner, J. M., "Trend towards earlier menarche in London, Oslo, Copenhagen, the Netherlands, and Hungary," *Nature* 1973; 243: 75–76.

Thrash, Agatha, M.D., *The Animal Connection*, Alabama: Yuchi Pines Institute, 1980.

———., *Eat For Strength: A Vegetarian Cookbook, Oil-Free*, Alabama: Thrash Publications, 1978.

Tock, B., Lanza, E., and Greenwald, P., "Dietary Fiber, Vegetables, and Colon Cancer: Critical Review and Meta-analyses of the Epidemiologic Evidence," *Journal of the National Cancer Institute* 1990; 82: 650–661.

Toniolo, Paolo, et al., "Calorie-Providing Nutrients and Risk of Breast Cancer," *Journal of the National Cancer Institute* 1989; 81: 278–286.

Toufexis, A., "Red Alert on Red Meat," *Time* magazine, December 24, 1990.

Troll, W., "Blocking of Tumor Promotion by Protease Inhibitors," in J. H. Burchenal and H. F. Oettgen, eds., *Cancer: Achievements, Challenges, and Prospects for the 1980's, Vol. 1*, New York: Grune and Stratton, 1980.

Truswell, A., "ABC of Nutrition. Reducing the risk of coronary heart disease," *British Medical Journal* 1985; 291: 34.

"Unrecognized Disorders Frequently Occurring Among Infants and Children from the Ill Effects of Milk," *Southern Medical Journal* September 1938; 31: 1016.

Vegan Outreach newsletter, June 1, 1998.

Vegetarian Journal, January–February 1998, Vol. XVII, No. 1.

Vegetarian Voice, Winter 1998, Vol. 22, No. 4.

Veggie Life, July 1998.

Viikari, J., "Multicenter study of atherosclerosis precursors in Finnish children: pilot study of 8-year old boys," *Annals of Clinical Research* 1982; 14: 103.

Wagman, Richard, M.D., F.A.C.P., ed. *The New Complete Medical and Health Encyclopedia,* Chicago: J. G. Ferguson Publishing Company: 1987.

Walker, A., "Osteoporosis and Calcium Deficiency," *American Journal of Clinical Nutrition* 1965; 16: 327.

Wattenberg, L. W., et al., *Cancer Prevention,* Boca Raton: CRC Press, 1992.

"What Causes Cancer on the Farm?" *Medical World News,* January 14, 1972; 39.

"Will eating less fat lower breast cancer risk after all?" *Tufts University Diet & Nutrition Letter,* 14:2, 1996.

Willett, Walter C., et al., "Relation of Meat, Fat, and Fiber Intake to the Risk of Colon Cancer in a Prospective Study Among Women," *New England Journal of Medicine* 1990; 323: 1664–1672.

World Health Organization, *Report of the Joint WHO/FAO Expert Consultation on Diet, Nutrition and the Prevention of Chronic Diseases,* Geneva, Switzerland, 2002

Wynder, E. L., Fujita, Y., Harris, R. E., and Hirayama, T., "Comparative epidemiology of cancer between the United States and Japan," *Cancer* 1991; 67: 746–763.

Yetiv, Jack, M.D., Ph.D., *Popular Nutritional Practices: A Scientific Appraisal,* Toledo, Ohio: Popular Medicine Press, 1986.

Ziegler, E. E., Fomon, S. J., Nelson, S. E., et al., "Cow milk feeding in infancy: further observations on blood loss from the gastrointestinal tract," *Journal of Pediatrics* 1990; 116: 11–18.

Appendix One

✠

THE PCRM DIET

(Modified from *New Four Food Groups*,
Physicians Committee for Responsible Medicine)

Now We Know

Many of us grew up with the USDA's old Basic Four Food Groups, first introduced in 1956. Since that time, we have learned about the importance of fiber, phytonutrients, and antioxidants, and the health risks of cholesterol and fats. We have also discovered that the plant kingdom provides excellent sources of nutrients once associated only with meat and dairy products—like protein, iron, and calcium. The USDA revised its recommendations in 1992 with the Food Guide Pyramid, a food grouping plan that reduced the serving suggestions for animal products and vegetable fats.

The Physicians Committee for Responsible Medicine (PCRM), however, realizing that regular consumption of such foods—even in lower quantities—poses serious, unnecessary health risks, had already developed the New Four Food Groups in 1991. The PCRM no-cholesterol, low-fat plan supplies all of an average adult's daily nutritional requirements, including substantial amounts of fiber. Heart disease, cancer, stroke, diabetes, high blood pressure, and obesity all have a dramatically lower average incidence among people consuming primarily plant-based diets. Try the New Four Food Groups and discover a healthier way to live!

What to Eat

- **Vegetables—3 or more servings a day**

  Vegetables are packed with nutrients; they provide vitamin C, beta-carotene, riboflavin, iron, calcium, fiber, and other nutrients. Dark green leafy vegetables, such as broccoli, collards, kale, mustard and turnip greens, chicory, and bok choy are especially good sources of these important nutrients. Dark yellow and orange vegetables, such as carrots, winter squash, sweet potatoes, and pumpkin, provide extra beta-carotene. Include generous portions of a variety of vegetables in your diet.

  Serving size: 1 cup raw vegetables; 1/2 cup cooked vegetables

- **Whole Grains—5 or more servings a day**

  This group includes bread, rice, pasta, hot or cold cereal, corn, oats, millet, barley, bulghur, buckwheat groats, quinoa, and tortillas. Build each of your meals around a hearty grain dish—grains are rich in fiber and other complex carbohydrates, as well as protein, B vitamins and zinc.

  Serving size: 1/2 cup hot cereal; 1 ounce dry cereal; 1 slice bread

- **Fruit—3 or more servings a day**

  Fruits are rich in fiber, vitamin C, and beta-carotene. Be sure to include at least one serving each day of fruits that are high in vitamin C; citrus fruits, melons, and strawberries are all good choices. Choose whole fruit over fruit juices, which do not contain very much fiber.

  Serving size: 1 medium piece of fruit; 1/2 cup cooked fruit; 4 ounces juice

- **Legumes—2 or more servings a day**

  Legumes, such as beans, peas, and lentils—are all good sources of fiber, protein, iron, calcium, zinc, and B vitamins. This group also includes chick peas, baked and refried beans, soy milk, tempeh, and texturized vegetable protein.

Serving size: 1/2 cup cooked beans; 4 ounces tofu or tempeh; 8 ounces soy milk

Remember: Reach for whole, fresh, raw, and organic produce whenever possible. Be sure to also include a good source of vitamin B12, such as fortified cereal or soy, rice, almond, or veggie milk, or vitamin supplements.

For more information, contact the Physicians Committee for Responsible Medicine at (202) 686-2210, or at www.pcrm.org. The American Medical Association recommends that you make changes to your current lifestyle regimen with the consultation of your physician. This information is not meant to replace the medical counsel of your doctor or individual consultation with a registered dietitian. Your health care provider and local health department can also be good resources for information on alcohol, tobacco, and other drugs. It is wise to keep yourself educated about health and seek reputable resources when considering changes to your current food and fitness lifestyle.

©Kerrie Saunders, *The Vegan Diet as Chronic Disease Prevention*, New York: Lantern Books, 2003

Appendix Two

⁜

FAMILY RESOURCE LIST
Be sure to ask your health care provider for helpful organizations in your area.

Books
Becoming Vegan by Brenda Davis, R.D. and Vesanto Melina, R.D.
Diet for a New America by John Robbins
Dr. Spock's Baby and Child Care, 7th ed. by Benjamin Spock, M.D.
Eat to Live by Joel Fuhrman, M.D.
Food for Life by Neal Barnard, M.D.
McDougall's Medicine: A Challenging Second Opinion by John McDougall, M.D.
New Vegetarian Baby by Sharon Yntema and Christine Beard
Pregnancy, Children, and the Vegan Diet by Michael Klaper, M.D.
Raising Vegetarian Children: A Guide to Good Health and Family Harmony by Joanne Stepaniak, Vesanto Melina, R.D.
A Vegetarian Doctor Speaks Out by Charles Attwood, M.D., F.A.A.P.
Vegetarian Pregnancy by Sharon Yntema

Magazines
Good Medicine (www.pcrm.org/magazine)
Satya (www.satyamag.com)
Veggie Life (www.veggielife.com)
VegNews (www.vegnews.com)
Vegetarian Voice (www.navs-online.org/voice/voice.html)
Vegetarian Journal (www.vrg.org/journal)

Organizations

International Lactation Consultant Association, (312) 541-1710

LaLeche League International, (800) 525-3243

National Alliance for Breastfeeding Advocacy, (410) 995-3726

Physicians Committee for Responsible Medicine, (202) 686-2210

Websites

www.americanvegan.org (The American Vegan Society: events, books, videos)

www.drfuhrman.com (Dr. Joel Fuhrman)

www.drklaper.com (Dr. Michael Klaper)

www.drmcdougall.com (Dr. John McDougall)

www.navs-online.org (North American Vegetarian Society, conferences, information)

www.pcrm.org (Physicians Committee for Responsible Medicine)

www.veganmd.org (Dr. Michael Greger)

www.vegetarianbaby.com (Vegetarian and vegan parents' online database)

www.vegsource.com (Support, information, cookbooks, experts)

www.vegfamily.com (Discussion boards, e-zine, recipes, support, information)

www.vrg.org (Vegetarian Resource Group, recipes, support, *Vegetarian Journal*)

APPENDIX THREE

✠

FACT SHEETS

ARTHRITIS AND DIET

Arthritis is a family of over 100 related diseases, including osteoarthritis, ankylosing spondylitis, gout, lupus, and rheumatoid arthritis. The various forms usually share the symptoms of inflammation, heat, swelling, stiffness, redness, pain, and degeneration. Other related conditions and symptoms include night sweats, dehydration, fatigue, dry eyes, gluten sensitivity, Chronic Fatigue Syndrome, gastritis, Leaky Gut Syndrome, weak immunity, and dysfunction of the thyroid, adrenal, or thymus glands.

The pain of arthritis is the end result of a normal process gone awry. When an area of the body has damage or infection, several different forms of white blood cells rush to the area to seek out the invading antigens, dissolve the invader, and then make repairs. In arthritis, however, the white blood cells also begin to digest cartilage, bone, ligament, muscle, or other tissues.

Getting Arthritis under Control

While the symptoms of arthritis can sometimes be managed by prescriptions, a change in diet and lifestyle can be a great help, maybe even eliminating the need for pain medication. Current theories on the ultimate culprit in arthritis include food allergies (especially to dairy products), acidity imbalance likely related to harm from excess animal proteins, and other processes whereby foreign antigens slip through the intestinal wall and into the bloodstream. Common trigger foods are listed below, and you can work with your doctor and/or dietitian to find out what to avoid, based on your own body's response to various foods. Doctors and dietitians trained in elimination diets can be of particular help. Learning to avoid your particular arthritis trigger foods can make a significant difference in the amount of pain you experience, and help stop the degenerative process.

In general, be sure to drink a minimum of five glasses of water daily to help with detoxification, learn to manage stress, and avoid your trigger foods. Many preventive medicine specialists now recommend a low-fat, high-fiber vegetarian diet to help alleviate

FOOD SOURCES TO CONSIDER AS TRIGGERS FOR YOUR ARTHRITIS

Animal flesh (beef, pork, bacon, lamb, fish, seafood, liver, brain, giz-
zards, chicken, turkey, venison, etc.)
Animal fluids (cow milk, butter, cheese, cottage cheese, ice cream,
yogurt, goat milk, etc.)

Coffee (caffeinated & decaffeinated	Grapefruit	Rye
	Malt	Sugar
Corn	Oats	Tea
Eggs (caviar, chicken eggs, etc.)	Oranges	Tomato
	Peanuts	Wheat

arthritic pain. This diet automatically eliminates most of the major offenders—like the proteins found in animal flesh and fluids (milk, cheese, beef, pork, chicken, lamb, bacon, etc.)—foods that also contribute dietary cholesterol and saturated fat. Research cited on arthritis in the *Lancet* (1991), the *American Journal of Clinical Nutrition* (1999), and the *British Journal of Rheumatology* (1997) supports the switch to such a diet for arthritis sufferers. A well-planned vegan diet also provides nutrients sometimes found to be low in arthritis sufferers, like omega-3 fatty acids, B5, B6, zinc, boron, selenium, manganese, and copper.

More Information on the Optimal Diet for Disease Prevention

Eating for maximum disease prevention means increasing the vita-mins, minerals, fiber, antioxidants, and phytonutrients in your diet, while reducing the hormones, antibiotics, cholesterol, saturated fat, excess protein, and concentrated pesticide content normally found in the Standard American Diet. Many physicians and dietitians are now aware of the benefits of proper lifestyle, exercise, and nutri-tion. The Physicians Committee for Responsible Medicine, Dean Ornish, M.D., Brenda Davis, R.D., Vesanto Melina, R.D., John McDougall, M.D., Joel Fuhrman, M.D., William Harris, M.D., and

Michael Klaper, M.D., are all wonderful resources for the health benefits of a low-fat, high-fiber vegetarian diet. Work with your doctor and enjoy your new health!

For more information, contact the Physicians Committee for Responsible Medicine at (202) 686-2210, or at www.pcrm.org. The American Medical Association recommends that you make changes to your current lifestyle regimen with the consultation of your physician. This information is not meant to replace the medical counsel of your doctor or individual consultation with a registered dietitian. Your health care provider and local health department can also be good resources for information on alcohol, tobacco, and other drugs. It is wise to keep yourself educated about health and seek reputable resources when considering changes to your current food and fitness lifestyle.

THE B VITAMINS

Properties, Benefits, and Healthy Sources

The B vitamins (also called B1, 2, 3, 5, 6, 12, 15, 17, B complex, thiamine, riboflavin, niacin, pantothenic acid, pyridoxine, cyanocobalamin, pangamic acid, amygdalin, biotin, choline, inositol, PABA, para-aminobenzoic acid, and folic acid) are used for many functions in the body. They help with immunity, pregnancy, lactation, food metabolism, handling stress, growth and development, detoxification, hormone function, electrolyte balance, and energy level maintenance. They are vital to nerve, organ, tissue, blood, gland, cell, and bone health. The B vitamins also help in the fight against cancer.

The best overall source of B vitamins, except for B12, discussed below, is from plant foods like fruits, vegetables, grains, beans, lentils, nuts, and seeds. Go for variety, and choose whole, fresh, organic produce as often as you can. Since some B vitamins are destroyed by heat, reach for raw fruits and vegetables whenever possible.

Vitamin B12 is made by bacteria and can be found in tiny amounts in our saliva, in the liver's bile, and in the intestines, but nutrition experts caution not to rely on these sources, or on the often-quoted statement that our liver stores B12 for three to five years, to meet our B12 needs. Animals typically accumulate B12 in their flesh or milk by consuming manure, commercial feed, water, and B12-rich soil. However, the use of synthetic herbicides, pesticides, and other chemicals that have a sterilizing effect on soil and plants has all but eliminated natural, plant-based foods as a reliable source of this bacteria-driven nutrient, and the similar effects of pasteurization, irradiation, and other processing methods suggest that even those who eat animal flesh or drink animal milk should ensure adequate B12 from fortified foods or supplements. Many of today's prepared vegan foods and veggie, soy, rice, or almond milks are fortified with B12, as are other soy products, cereals, and Red Star Vegetarian Support Formula Nutritional Yeast, making this important issue easier to address.

Symptoms of Low B
Common symptoms of B-vitamin deficiency include fatigue, muscle pain, hair loss, high blood pressure, high cholesterol, irritability, poor concentration, memory loss, poor growth in children, and skin conditions.

Too Much B
If you take excessive vitamin B supplements, to the point of toxicity, you may experience side effects. Although toxicity is rare, diarrhea, dizziness, liver trouble, nausea, depression, and flushing are examples of symptoms that may occur.

About Supplements
As a general rule, the B vitamins work best in a balance, so be sure to work with your doctor to avoid problems with supplementation. For example, excess B6 can interfere with levodopa prescriptions. Natural, whole, and unrefined plant food sources (listed below) are your best bet for overall health and prevention of nutrient deficiency. Whole foods contain vitamins, minerals, fiber, protein, fat, carbohydrate, and phytonutrients in a wonderful variety of balanced combinations. If you or your doctor is considering a nutrient supplement or prescription, always work together (or with a dietitian) to determine the correct dose. Try to take B vitamin supplements with foods that also contain these vitamins, to help your body better absorb the nutrients. Remember—if you have a kidney, liver, or digestive ailment, or other serious illness, you will need to be especially careful with supplementation.

For more information, contact the Physicians Committee for Responsible Medicine at (202) 686-2210, or at www.pcrm.org. The American Medical Association recommends that you make changes to your current lifestyle regimen with the consultation of your physician. This information is not meant to replace the medical counsel of your doctor or individual consultation with a registered dietitian. Your health care provider and local health department can also be good resources for information on alcohol, tobacco, and other drugs. It is wise to keep yourself educated about health and seek reputable resources when considering changes to your current food and fitness lifestyle.

FOOD SOURCES FOR B VITAMINS

Alfalfa	Hazelnuts	Pumpkin seeds
Almonds	Juniper berries	Raisins
Apple	Kale	Seeds
Apricot	Kelp	Sesame seeds
Asparagus	Lemon	Soybeans
Avocado	Leafy greens	Spinach
Banana	Lentils	Spirulina
Barley	Lima beans	Sprouts
Beans	Lettuce	Strawberries
Beets	Melons	Sunflower seeds
Bell peppers	Millet	Tomato
Black-eyed peas	Mung beans	Unrefined molasses
Broccoli	Mushrooms	Wheat
Brown rice	Navy beans	Wheatgrass
Bulghur	Northern beans	Wild rice
Cabbage	Oats	Watercress
Cantaloupe	Oatmeal	Walnuts
Carrot	Okra	Wheat bran
Cashews	Onion	Wheat germ
Cauliflower	Orange	Yellow fruits
Celery	Papaya	
Cherries	Parsley	
Corn	Peaches	Fortified hot or cold
Cucumber	Peas	cereals, and soy, rice,
Dates	Peanuts	almond, or veggie
Dulse	Pears	milks. Nutritional
Figs	Pecans	yeast containing
Flax seeds	Persimmon	cobalamin/cyanoco-
Garbanzo beans	Pineapple	balamin
Garlic	Potato	
Green vegetables	Prunes	

BUILDING BETTER BONES

The Healing Process of a Broken Bone

The process of healing a broken bone is very similar to the healing process of skin. As soon as a bone breaks, a jacket of cells forms around the break, in the same way skin forms a scab of cells around broken skin. Unfortunately, the callus only protects from infections, and further damage can be done if it is not kept in a cast. The cast that your doctor applies will keep the bone straight while it heals. Whenever possible, the cast will be set in such a way that you are still able to use it, because bone and muscle grow when used.

Osteoporosis

Osteoporosis is a condition of brittle bones that contributes to an abnormal and unhealthy loss of bone calcium into the urine. Both men and women can suffer from this disease, which can lead to fractures, infections, surgeries, and hospitalizations. Osteopoenia and osteomalacia are often the precursors to osteoporosis.

Product advertisers usually present the cause of osteoporosis as a lack of dietary calcium, and then market cows' milk as the best prevention. However, many nutrition experts agree that "this is not supported by the most recent comprehensive analysis of studies looking at dairy intake and bone health," as stated regarding women in the *American Journal of Clinical Nutrition*. The authors add, "There are two few studies in males and minority ethnic groups to determine whether dairy foods promote bone health in most of the U.S. population."[1] A 1994 study in the *American Journal of Epidemiology* on elderly men and women in Australia showed that higher dairy product consumption was associated with *increased* fracture risk. Those with the highest dairy product consumption had approximately double the risk of hip fracture compared to those with the lowest consumption. And, as Walter Willett, M.D., of Harvard University, points out, there are at least five good reasons to avoid dairy foods: "lactose intolerance, saturated fat, extra calories, possible increased risk of prostate cancer and ovarian cancer."[2] By controlling basic factors, you can have an enormous influence on whether calcium stays in your bones or drains out of your body.

Our bones are actually made of living tissue, breaking down and rebuilding continuously. Since the bones are alive, the process of osteoporosis can often be prevented or reversed, especially if action is taken early on. If you already have osteoporosis, talk with your doctor about exercises and perhaps even medications that can reverse it.

Hormone Supplements and Osteoporosis

Some doctors recommend estrogen supplements for women after menopause as a way to slow osteoporosis, although the effect is not very great over the long run, and hormones are rarely able to stop or reverse bone loss. Many women find these hormones distasteful because the most commonly prescribed brand, Premarin, is made from pregnant mares' urine, as its name suggests. What has many physicians worried is the fact that estrogens increase the risk of breast cancer. The Harvard Nurses' Health Study found that women taking estrogens have 30–80% more breast cancer compared to other women. For more information on other risks, including heart disease, blood clots, and gallbladder disease, contact the Physicians Committee for Responsible Medicine. Controlling calcium losses is a much safer strategy.

Factors in Bone Density Loss

Animal proteins tend to leach much more calcium from our bones than do plant proteins. Excess caffeine or sodium (salt) in your diet can also greatly increase the calcium loss through your kidneys. If you reduce your total sodium intake to 1–2 grams per day, your bones will be able to hold onto their calcium much better. So try avoiding salty snack foods, canned goods with added sodium, and avoid or lower the amount of salt you use at the stove and table to a minimum. Alcohol can weaken your bones, apparently by reducing the body's ability to make new bone to replace normal losses. The effect is probably only significant if you have more than two drinks per day of spirits, beer, or wine.

Smokers tend to have a 40% higher risk of bone fractures than non-smokers, as shown in an identical twin study cited in 1994 in the *New England Journal of Medicine*. A lower than normal amount of testosterone can encourage osteoporosis, and about 40% of men over 70 years of age have decreased levels of testosterone. Steroid medications, such as prednisone, are a common cause of bone loss and fractures. If you are receiving steroids, you will want to work with your doctor to minimize the dose and to explore other treatments.

The Best Prevention: Exercise and the PCRM Diet

A variety of "weight-bearing" exercises will also help prevent osteoporosis. Research shows that sedentary people lose calcium, while active people who stimulate and use their bones and muscles retain a much healthier bone density. Exercises like walking, dancing, yoga, non-impact aerobics, tennis, racquetball, and weightlifting are wonderful ways to increase your bone density.

Based on international and cross-cultural studies, the best diet for the prevention of osteoporosis is a well-balanced, low-fat, high-fiber vegetarian diet, which eliminates the animal protein implicated in the loss of calcium from bones. It seems that the acidity required for humans to digest animal flesh and fluids needs an alkaline buffer—which the body makes by taking calcium from the bones. Dairy products do contain calcium, but it is accompanied by animal proteins, lactose sugar, animal growth factors, occasional drugs and contaminants, and a substantial amount of fat and cholesterol in all but the defatted versions. The Physicians Committee for Responsible Medicine diet is ideal for the prevention of osteoporosis and many of its related problems. The most healthful calcium sources are "greens and beans"—green leafy vegetables and legumes. The main exceptions are spinach, Swiss chard, and beet greens, which contain a large amount of calcium but tend to hold onto it very tenaciously, so that you will absorb less of it. Many healthful calcium sources are listed below.

About Supplements

The body uses a variety of materials to build and maintain bones, including calcium, phosphorus, protein, hormones, collagen, boron, manganese, silicon, and magnesium, just to name a few. If you are considering calcium or vitamin D supplementation, work with your physician. Non-elderly, light-skinned individuals in sunny climates (like Los Angeles or Atlanta and farther south) can usually get enough sunlight to make adequate vitamin D with about fifteen minutes of midmorning or afternoon sunlight per day on the face or forearms. Darker skin requires three to six times more sunlight than lighter skin to produce the same amount of vitamin D (with the darkest skin requiring the longest exposure), because in a given period less sunlight reaches the deeper layers of darker skin. For those who do not get sufficient sunlight (including those who wear sunscreen or live in less sunny climates), or who are elderly

FOOD SOURCES OF CALCIUM

Agar	Carrots	Pinto beans
Almond butter	Chick peas	Pistachios
Almonds	Collard greens	Raisins
Amaranth	Figs	Sesame seeds
Barley	Garbanzo beans	Soybeans
Black turtle beans	Great northern beans	Sunflower seeds
Blackstrap molasses	Green beans	Sweet potatoes
Bok choy	Hazelnuts	Tempeh
Brazil nuts	Kale	Tofu with calcium
Broccoli	Kidney beans	Turnip greens
Brussels sprouts	Lentils	Vegetarian baked
Butternut squash	Mustard greens	beans
Calcium-fortified	Navy beans	White beans
almond, soy, veg-	Oatmeal	Yellow beans
gie, or rice milks	Okra	
Calcium-fortified	Oranges	
orange juice	Parsley	

with a reduced capacity to synthesize vitamin D, fortified foods or supplements can be used to ensure adequate vitamin D.

Natural, whole, and unrefined plant food sources are your best bet for overall health and prevention of nutrient deficiency. Whole foods contain vitamins, minerals, fiber, protein, fat, carbohydrate, and phytonutrients in a wonderful variety of balanced combinations. If you are considering a nutrient supplement or prescription, always work together with your doctor (or with a dietitian) to determine the correct dose. Try to take supplements with a food that contains the nutrient to help your body better absorb and use it. Remember—if you have a kidney, liver, or digestive ailment, or other serious illness, you will need to be especially careful with supplementation.

References
1.   Weinsier R. L., Krumdieck C. L., "Dairy foods and bone health: examination of the evidence," *American Journal of Clinical Nutrition* 2000 72(3) 681–9; 2001 73(3) 660, 661.
2.   Willett, Walter, M.D., Ph.D., *Eat, Drink and Be Healthy: The Harvard Medical School Guide to Healthy Eating* (New York: Simon and Schuster, 2001), 144.

For more information, contact the Physicians Committee for Responsible Medicine at (202) 686-2210, or at www.pcrm.org. The American Medical Association recommends that you make changes to your current lifestyle regimen with the consultation of your physician. This information is not meant to replace the medical counsel of your doctor or individual consultation with a registered dietitian. Your health care provider and local health department can also be good resources for information on alcohol, tobacco, and other drugs. It is wise to keep yourself educated about health and seek reputable resources when considering changes to your current food and fitness lifestyle.
© Kerrie Saunders, *The Vegan Diet as Chronic Disease Prevention*, New York: Lantern Books, 2003

CANCER AND DIET
(Modified from *Foods for Cancer Prevention*,
Physicians Committee for Responsible Medicine)

What Is Cancer?
Cancer begins as a single abnormal cell that begins to multiply out of control. Groups of such cells form tumors and invade healthy tissue, often spreading to other parts of the body. Carcinogens are substances that promote the development of cancerous cells. They may come from foods, from the air, or even from within the body. Most carcinogens are neutralized before damage can occur, but sometimes they attack the cell's genetic material (DNA) and alter it. It takes years for a noticeable tumor to develop. During this time, compounds known as *inhibitors* can keep the cells from growing. Some vitamins in plant foods are known to be inhibitors. Dietary fat, on the other hand, is known to be a promoter that helps the abnormal cells grow quickly.

Of the many diseases that affect people these days, cancer is among the most feared. But despite a wealth of scientific data, most people remain unaware of how they can reduce their risk of developing cancer. According to the National Cancer Institute, as much as 80% of all cancers are due to identified factors, and thus are potentially preventable. Excessive intake of alcohol raises one's risks for cancers of the breast, mouth, pharynx, and esophagus. When smoking is added to the picture, these risks skyrocket, along with risks of stomach, liver, and colon cancers. Thirty percent of cancers are caused by tobacco use, and as much as 35–50% are caused by diet.

How Fat Affects Cancer Risks
Fat increases hormone production and thus raises breast cancer risks. It also stimulates the production of bile acids, which have been linked to colon cancer. The average diet in the U.S. is about 37% fat. The National Cancer Institute suggests that people lower that percentage down to 30%, and many preventive medicine physicians recommend going lower.

Although the total amount of fat one eats is of concern, we now know that saturated fats, animal fats, and trans fats cause harm, and monounsaturated fats like olive oil can actually have a protective effect. One study noted a 200% increase in breast cancer among those who consume beef or pork five to six times per week. Dr. Sheila Bingham, a prominent cancer researcher from the University of Cambridge, notes that meat is more closely associated with colon cancer than any other factor.[1] Meat and milk are also linked to both prostate and ovarian cancers.[2]

Cross-cultural studies have revealed that the populations with the highest levels of fat consumption are also the ones with the highest death rates from breast and colon cancer. The lowest rates are in groups with the lowest consumption of fats.[3] Migration studies help to rule out the influence of genetics.[4] Many studies indicate that fat in foods increases one's risk for cancer, and may also adversely affect breast cancer survival rates for those who have cancer.[5]

Fiber Fights Cancer

In 1970, British physician Dennis Burkitt observed that a high-fiber diet reduces diseases of the digestive tract. He noted that in countries where diets are high in fiber (that is, plant-based diets), there were fewer cases of colon cancer. His findings hold true all over the world, as nations whose diets are based upon animal products— like the United States—have the highest rates of colon cancer. Animal products contain no fiber.

Fiber cannot be digested by humans early in the digestive process; instead it works to move food more quickly through the intestines, helping to eliminate carcinogens. It also draws water into the digestive tract. The water and fiber make fecal matter bulkier, so carcinogens are diluted. Bile acids are secreted into the intestine to help digest fat; there, bacteria can change the acids into chemicals, which promote colon cancer. Fiber may bind with these bile acids and evict them from the intestines.[6]

Fiber is also protective against other forms of cancer. Studies have shown that stomach cancer and breast cancer are less common on high-fiber diets.[7,8] Fiber helps to keep hormones like estrogen in balance, too, which is important for the prevention of breast cancer. Estrogens are normally secreted into the intestine, where the fiber binds with the hormone and moves it out of the body.[9] Without adequate fiber, the estrogen can be reabsorbed from the intestine into the bloodstream. High levels of estrogen are linked to a higher risk of breast cancer.

Most Americans average about 10–20 grams of fiber a day, but experts recommend 30–40 grams per day. The best sources of fiber are whole grains, beans, peas, lentils, fruits, and vegetables. Foods that are closest to their natural state, unrefined and unpeeled, are highest in fiber. Excessive intake of alcohol raises one's risks for cancers of the breast, mouth, pharynx, and esophagus. When combined with smoking, these risks skyrocket. It also raises risks for stomach, liver, and colon cancers.[10]

The Importance of Vegetables

The evidence points to a diet that is plant-based, low in fat (especially trans fats, animal fats, and saturated fat), and high in fiber, including a variety of fruits, vegetables, whole grains, and beans, for chronic disease prevention. Vegetables are not only low in fat and high in fiber, but also contain many cancer-fighting substances. Vegetarians have stronger immune systems and higher blood levels of beta-carotene than meat eaters, and they consume more vitamin C, beta-carotene, indoles, and fiber. Vegetarians have about half the cancer risk of meat eaters.[11] German researchers also discovered recently that vegetarians have more than twice the natural killer cell activity (natural killer cells are specialized white blood cells that attack and neutralize cancer cells) of meat eaters.[12] A diet that is rich in soybeans may be one reason for the lower incidence of breast cancer in Asia. Carotenoids, the pigment that gives fruits and vegetables their dark colors, have been shown to help prevent cancer. Beta-carotene, present in dark green and yellow vegetables, helps protect against lung cancer and may help prevent cancers of the bladder, mouth, larynx, esophagus, breast, and other sites. Vegetables such as cabbage, broccoli, kale, turnips, cauliflower, and

Brussels sprouts contain flavones and indoles, which are thought to have anti-cancer activities.

Vitamin C, found in citrus fruits and many vegetables, may lower risks for cancers of the esophagus and stomach. This vitamin acts as an antioxidant, neutralizing cancer-causing chemicals that form in the body. It also blocks the conversion of nitrates to cancer-causing nitrosamines in the stomach. Selenium is found in whole grains and has antioxidant effects similar to those of vitamin C, vitamin E, and beta-carotene. If you are considering a nutrient supplement or prescription, always work with your doctor (or with a dietitian) to determine the correct dose and avoid potential risks. Remember—if you have a kidney, liver, or digestive ailment, or other serious illness, you will need to be especially careful with supplementation.

References

1. Bingham S. A., "Meat, starch, and non-starch polysaccharides and bowel cancer," *American Journal of Clinical Nutrition* 1988; 48: 762–7.

2. Rose D. P., Boyar A. P., Wynder E. L., "International comparisons of mortality rates for cancer of the breast, ovary, prostate, and colon, and per capita food consumption," *Cancer* 1986; 58: 2363–71.

3. Lan H. W., Carpenter J. T., "Breast cancer: incidence, nutritional concerns, and treatment approaches," *Journal of the American Dietetic Association* 1987; 87: 765–9.

4. Minowa M., Bingham S., Cummings J. H., "Dietary fiber intake in Japan," *Human Nutrition. Applied Nutrition* 1983; 37A: 113–9.

5. Wynder E. L., Rose D. P., Cohen L. A., "Diet and breast cancer in causation and therapy," *Cancer* 1986; 58: 1804–13.

6. Kritchevsky D., "Diet, nutrition, and cancer: the role of fiber," *Cancer* 1986; 58: 1830–6.

7. Risch H. A., Jain M., Choi N. W., et al., "Dietary factors and the incidence of cancer of the stomach," *American Journal of Epidemiology* 1985; 122: 947–59.

8. Lubin F, Wax Y., Modan B., et al., "Role of fat, animal protein and dietary fiber in breast cancer etiology: a case control study," *Journal of the National Cancer Institute* 1986; 77: 605–12.

9. Goldin B. R., Adlercreutz H., Gorbach S. L., et al., "Estrogen excretion patterns and plasma levels in vegetarian and omnivorous women," *New England Journal of Medicine* 1982; 307: 1542–7.

10. Breslow N. E., Enstrom J. E., "Geographic correlations between cancer mortality rates and alcohol-tobacco consumption in the United States," *Journal of the National Cancer Institute* 1974; 53: 631–9.

11. Phillips R. L., "Role of lifestyle and dietary habits in risk of cancer among Seventh-day Adventists," *Cancer Research* 1975; 35(Suppl): 3513–22.

12. Malter M., "Natural killer cells, vitamins, and other blood components of vegetarian and omnivorous men," *Nutrition and Cancer* 1989; 12: 271–8.

For more information, contact the Physicians Committee for Responsible Medicine at (202) 686-2210, or at www.pcrm.org. The American Medical Association recommends that you make changes to your current lifestyle regimen with the consultation of your physician. This information is not meant to replace the medical counsel of your doctor or individual consultation with a registered dietitian. Your health care provider and local health department can also be good resources for information on alcohol, tobacco, and other drugs. It is wise to keep yourself educated about health and seek reputable resources when considering changes to your current food and fitness lifestyle.

© Kerrie Saunders, *The Vegan Diet as Chronic Disease Prevention*, New York: Lantern Books, 2003

CHOLESTEROL, STROKE, AND HEART DISEASE
(Modified from *Cholesterol and Heart Disease*,
Physicians Committee for Responsible Medicine)

A Family of Related Diseases

When blood circulation is disrupted, damage can occur anywhere in the body. If the blood supply to the heart is lost, we call it a heart attack. If the blood to the brain is lost, we call it a stroke. We can also experience decreased circulation elsewhere in the body, causing symptoms such as impotence, hair loss, vision loss, hearing loss, and loss of feeling.

Every day, more than 4,000 Americans suffer a heart attack. Those who survive often go on to have another one. But this need not happen. Eating habits and other parts of our lifestyle play a large role in the risk of heart disease. The good news is that heart disease can usually be prevented and even reversed.

Atherosclerosis is the all-too-common form of heart disease in which plaques of cholesterol and other substances, very much like small tumors, form in the artery walls. Eventually, the passageway for blood becomes clogged. Less blood flow means less oxygen for the heart muscle. Chest pain (angina) occurs, usually following exercise or excitement, but a heart attack occurs when a part of the heart muscle dies due to the cut-off blood supply.

Atherosclerosis is *not* caused by old age. When battlefield casualties were examined during the Korean and Vietnam wars, American soldiers had significant atherosclerosis at only 18 or 20 years of age. Their Asian counterparts, raised on a diet consisting mainly of rice and vegetables, had much healthier arteries. The main reason that older people are more likely to have heart problems than younger people is that they have had more time to indulge in unhealthy habits. Similarly, most people do not have a hereditary tendency toward heart disease. In most cases the problem is not usually due to genetics, but to eating habits and smoking. Your doctor can tell you if you belong to the 5% of the population with a true genetic tendency toward heart disease.

Many studies have shown the connection between cholesterol and heart problems. Beginning in 1949, under the direction of William Castelli, M.D., the population of Framingham, Massachusetts, has been monitored for thirty-five years to see which factors influence the rate of heart disease. Dr. Castelli concludes that there is a cholesterol level below which the risk of a heart attack is insignificant. According to Castelli, "Three quarters of the people who live on the face of this earth never have a heart attack. They live in Asia, Africa, and South America, and their cholesterols are all around 150."

What Is Cholesterol?
Cholesterol is more like a wax than a fat. The liver manufactures about 600–800 milligrams of cholesterol every day for the body to use in the manufacture of hormones and cell membranes, and in other parts of the body. Cholesterol levels are measured in milligrams (mg) of cholesterol per deciliter (dl) of blood serum. Based on the results of the Framingham Heart Study and other research, the ideal level appears to be below 150 mg/dl. At that point, a heart attack is very unlikely. Unfortunately, the average cholesterol level in America is 205, which is not far from the average level for heart attack victims (244). Surprisingly, the federal government's recommended maximum level is still as high as 200. For disease prevention, though, today's medical professionals should seek the ideal level of below 150 mg/dl.

When cholesterol is transported in the bloodstream, it is packed into low-density lipoproteins (LDL), sometimes called "bad cholesterol." Although LDL is necessary in limited quantities, a high LDL cholesterol level can dramatically increase your risk of a heart attack. LDL delivers cholesterol to various parts of the body. When cholesterol is released from dead cells, it is picked up for disposal in another kind of package, called high-density lipoproteins (HDL), the "good cholesterol." When doctors measure cholesterol levels, they first look at total cholesterol as a good, quick guide to a person's risk. For a more exact guide, they divide the total level by the HDL level. The lower your total cholesterol level, and the higher your HDL as a proportion of this, the lower your risk of a heart attack.

The ratio of total cholesterol to HDL should, ideally, be around 3 to 1. Unfortunately, the average American male's ratio is much higher than that, at 5.1 to 1. Vegetarians, on the other hand, average only about 2.9 to 1.[1] Smoking and obesity appear to lower HDL; eating foods rich in vitamin C increases it.[2]

How to Lower Your Cholesterol

We do not need to eat cholesterol, which is only found in animals and animal products. Every 100 mg of cholesterol in your daily diet—that is, every 4 ounces of beef or chicken, half an egg, or three cupts of milk—adds roughly five points to your cholesterol level, although this varies from person to person. Beef and chicken have the same amount of cholesterol, 25 mg per ounce.[3]

Plant foods, however, never contain cholesterol, so people can reduce their cholesterol levels dramatically by changing the foods they eat. Every time you reduce your cholesterol level by 1%, you reduce your risk of heart disease by 2%.[4] For example, a reduction from 300 mg/dl to 200 mg/dl (i.e., a one-third reduction) will yield a two-thirds reduction in the risk of a heart attack. For some people, the benefits are even greater.

Animal products also contain saturated fat, which causes the liver to produce more cholesterol. Unfortunately, the food industry often presents the fat content of certain products in a misleading way. By reporting the fat content by weight, they make these products look more healthful than they actually are. The important piece of information is the percentage of calories from fat. Even in the leanest cuts of beef, about 30% of the calories come from fat. Skinless chicken is nearly as high, at 23%. Even without the skin, chicken is never truly a low-fat food.

The percentage of calories from fat in grains, beans, vegetables, and fruits, however, is comfortably under 10%. The few vegetable oils that are high in fat are palm kernel oil, coconut oil, and hydrogenated oils. While liquid vegetable oils are much better than animal fats and tropical oils, all fats and oils are natural mixtures of saturated and unsaturated fats. Available research contends that olive oil and canola oil are our best choices for food preparation.

Learning to manage stress can really help, too.[5] Daily life is full of events that cause our hearts to beat a bit faster and drive up our blood pressure.[6] Reducing stress means keeping your challenges within a range you can manage. Getting adequate rest and learning techniques for stress reduction, meditation, or yoga can be very helpful. However, these measures cannot undo the effects of a bad diet. The only way to a healthy heart is an all-encompassing healthy lifestyle that incorporates a varied, low-fat, vegetarian diet, daily physical activity, and stress reduction.

Reversing Heart Disease

On July 21, 1990, the *Lancet* published the findings of Dean Ornish, M.D., who demonstrated that heart disease can actually be reversed without medicines.[7] Until then, most doctors were not even attempting to reverse heart disease, even though it was, as it is now, the most common cause of death. Most believed that the plaques of cholesterol and other substances that clog the arteries to the heart would not go away. The traditional way to remove them was to wait until they became severe enough to warrant a bypass or angioplasty.

At the University of California in San Francisco, Dr. Ornish tested the theory that a more potent diet, along with other lifestyle changes, might actually reverse heart disease. He selected patients who had plaques that were clearly visible on angiograms, and split the patients into two groups. Half were referred to a control group in which they received the standard care that doctors prescribe for heart patients. The other half began a vegetarian diet in which less than 10% of calories came from fat. They were also asked to begin a program of modest exercise, and learned to manage stress through a variety of simple techniques. Of course, smoking was not permitted.

Dr. Ornish's patients started to feel better almost immediately, and continued to improve over the course of the year. They had been struggling with the crushing chest pain of heart disease, but "most of them became essentially pain-free," Dr. Ornish said, "even though they were doing more activities, going back to work, and doing things that they hadn't been able to do, in some cases, for years." Not only did their cholesterol levels drop dramatically, but, after a year, 82% of the patients who followed Dr. Ornish's program showed measurable reversal of their coronary artery blockages. The plaques were starting to dissolve with no medications, no surgery, and no side effects. The control group, following the more traditional medical routine, did not do so well. For most patients, chest pain did not go away, but continued to get worse, and their plaques continued to grow, cutting off blood flow to the heart a bit more with every passing day. Dr. Ornish and other experts like Dr. Caldwell Esselstyn, a renowned cardiologist at the Cleveland Clinic, have "raised the bar" in the prevention and treatment of chronic disease.

Many doctors still recommend "chicken and fish" diets, even though a number of studies have shown that, in general, heart patients who make such moderate dietary changes tend to get worse over time. Those who adopt a low-fat, vegetarian diet, get daily physical activity, avoid tobacco, and manage stress, stand the best chance of reversing heart disease. We now have the most powerful tools yet for gaining control over the health of our hearts.

References
1. Castelli W. P., "Epidemiology of coronary heart disease," *American Journal of Medicine* 1984; 76(2A): 4–12.
2. Trout D. L., "Vitamin C and cardiovascular risk factors," *American Journal of Clinical Nutrition* 1991; 53: 322S–5S.
3. Pennington J. A. T., *Bowes and Church's Food Values of Portions Commonly Used*, New York: Harper and Row, 1989.
4. Lipid Research Clinics Program, "The Lipid Research Clinic's Coronary Primary Prevention Trial Results, II," *Journal of the American Medical Association* 1984; 251(3): 365–74.
5. Salonen J. T., Salonen R., Nyyssonen K., Korpela H., "Iron sufficiency is associated with hypertension and excess risk of myocardial infarction: the Kuopio Ischaemic Heart Disease Risk Factor Study (KIHD)," *Circulation* 1992; 85: 759–64.
6. Schnall P. L., Pieper C., Schwartz J. E., et al., "The relationship between 'job strain,' workplace diastolic blood pressure, and left ventricular mass index," *Journal of the American Medical Association* 1990; 263: 1929–35.

7.   Ornish D., Brown S. E., Scherwitz L. W., et al., "Can lifestyle changes reverse coronary heart disease?" *Lancet* 1990; 336: 129–33.

Suggested Reading
Foods That Fight Pain by Neal Barnard, M.D.
Eat Right, Live Longer by Neal Barnard, M.D.
Food for Life by Neal Barnard, M.D.
Dr. Dean Ornish's Program for Reversing Heart Disease by Dean Ornish, M.D.
The McDougall Plan by John McDougall, M.D.
The McDougall Program by John McDougall, M.D.

For more information, contact the Physicians Committee for Responsible Medicine at (202) 686-2210, or at www.pcrm.org. The American Medical Association recommends that you make changes to your current lifestyle regimen with the consultation of your physician. This information is not meant to replace the medical counsel of your doctor or individual consultation with a registered dietitian. Your health care provider and local health department can also be good resources for information on alcohol, tobacco, and other drugs. It is wise to keep yourself educated about health and seek reputable resources when considering changes to your current food and fitness lifestyle.
© Kerrie Saunders, *The Vegan Diet as Chronic Disease Prevention*, New York: Lantern Books, 2003

DIET AND DIABETES
(Slightly modified from *Diet and Diabetes*,
Physicians Committee for Responsible Medicine)

What Is Diabetes?

Diabetes is a condition in which the cells of the body cannot get the sugar they need. Glucose, a simple sugar, is the body's main fuel. It is present in the blood, but in diabetics it cannot get into the cells where it is needed. When diabetes starts in childhood (insulin-dependent diabetes), it is due to an inadequate supply of insulin, the hormone that ushers sugar into the cells of the body. Without insulin, the cell membranes keep sugar out. This form of diabetes is also called Type 1 or childhood-onset diabetes.

When diabetes begins in adulthood (non-insulin-dependent diabetes), it is not due to an inadequate supply of insulin. There is plenty of insulin in the bloodstream, but the cells do not respond readily to it. Sugar cannot easily get into the cells, and it backs up in the bloodstream. This form is also called Type 2 or adult-onset diabetes. In the short run, diabetics may experience episodes of labored breathing, vomiting, and dehydration. In the long run, diabetics are at risk for heart disease, kidney problems, disorders of vision, and other difficulties.

The Old Approach

The old approach to diabetes was to focus on restricting carbohydrates, like starches, breads, fruits, and refined sugars. The rationale was based on the fact that diabetics' urine contains sugar. Unfortunately, restricting carbohydrates can lead to a diet that is too high in protein and fat.

The New Approach

The new approach focuses more attention on fat. We have learned that the more fat there is in the diet, the harder time insulin has in getting sugar into the cell. Exactly why this occurs is not clear. But what is clear is that minimizing fat intake and reducing body fat help insulin do its job much better. Modern diabetic treatment programs drastically reduce meats, high-fat dairy products, and oils. At the same time, they increase grains, legumes, and vegetables. One study found that 21 of 23 patients on oral medications and 13 of 17 patients on insulin were able to stop their medications after 26 days on a near-vegetarian diet and exercise program.[1] During two-and three-year follow-ups, most diabetics treated with this regimen have retained their gains.[2] The dietary changes are simple, but profound, and they work. Low-fat, vegetarian diets are ideal for diabetics.

The second essential component to managing diabetes is exercise. Through regular exercise, the need for insulin injections can often be reduced, and oral medications often become unnecessary. This holds true not only for people with non-insulin-dependent diabetes, but also to some extent for those with insulin-dependent diabetes. Exercising muscles have a voracious appetite for fuel. When an individual is engaged in regular aerobic exercise, the sugar is able to enter the cells without the need for as much, or perhaps any, insulin. While people with non-insulin-dependent diabetes can often eliminate medications when their weight is reduced and foods and exercise are better controlled, those with insulin dependence will always need a source of insulin.

Questioning Cow Milk
The cause of insulin-dependent diabetes remains elusive. Several recent studies have implicated cow-milk consumption as a possible contributor.[3] When milk consumption patterns were examined across various nations, there was a very strong correlation with the incidence of insulin-dependent diabetes. It may be that milk proteins cause an autoimmune reaction in which the body mistakenly attacks its own insulin-producing cells.

Even so, a good diet and regular exercise can minimize the amount of insulin that insulin-dependent diabetics require. It is doubly important to keep fit and to keep dietary fat to a minimum, because diabetics are prone to heart disease and other blood vessel problems. However, the typical American Diabetes Association (ADA) diet contains about 300 milligrams of cholesterol per day and is about 30% fat. The fact is, diabetics are shortchanged by the diet most doctors give them. This fact sheet is not intended as a comprehensive program for diabetes. If you have diabetes, consult your doctor and tailor a program for your needs. But it is important to recognize that, for many, diabetes is a disease that need never occur. In most cases, diabetics can manage their disease much better with a food plan that gets most of its calories from complex carbohydrates while minimizing fats. At the same time, regular, vigorous exercise helps insulin work optimally.

References

1. Brand J. C., Snow B. J., Nabhan G. P., Truswell A. S., "Plasma glucose and insulin responses to traditional Pima Indian meals," *American Journal of Clinical Nutrition* 1990; 51(3): 416–20.
2. Barnard R. J., Massey M. R., Cherny S., O'Brien L.T., Pritikin N., "Long-term use of a high-complex-carbohydrate, highfiber, low-fat diet and exercise in the treatment of NIDDM patients," *Diabetes Care* 1983; 6(3): 268–73.
3. Scott F. W., "Cow milk and insulin-dependent diabetes mellitus: is there a relationship?" *American Journal of Clinical Nutrition* 1990; 51: 489–91.
    Karjalainen J., Martin J. M., Knip M., et al., "A bovine albumin peptide as a possible trigger of insulin-dependent diabetes mellitus," *New England Journal of Medicine* 1992; 327: 302–7.

Authors and Resources

American Dietetic Association Vegetarian Practice Group; Physicians Committee for Responsible Medicine; Charles Attwood, M.D.; Brenda Davis, R.D.; George Eisman, R.D.; Caldwell Esselstyn, M.D.; Joel Fuhrman, M.D.; William Harris, M.D.; Suzanne Havala, M.S., R.D., F.A.D.A.; Michael Klaper, M.D.; Reed Mangels, Ph.D., R.D., F.A.D.A.; John McDougall, M.D.; Vesanto Melina, M.S., R.D.; Dean Ornish, M.D.; Jennifer Raymond, R.D.; Virginia Messina, M.P.H., R.D.; Sharon Yntema, M.A.

For more information, contact the Physicians Committee for Responsible Medicine at (202) 686-2210, or at www.pcrm.org. The American Medical Association recommends that you make changes to your current lifestyle regimen with the consultation of your physician. This information is not meant to replace the medical counsel of your doctor or individual consultation with a registered dietitian. Your health care provider and local health department can also be good resources for information on alcohol, tobacco, and other drugs. It is wise to keep yourself educated about health and seek reputable resources when considering changes to your current food and fitness lifestyle.

© Kerrie Saunders, *The Vegan Diet as Chronic Disease Prevention*, New York: Lantern Books, 2003

ESSENTIAL FATTY ACIDS
(Properties, Benefits, and Healthy Sources)

Fatty acids (also called omega-3,-6,-9; EPA, DHA, ALA, SDA, LA, DGLA, AA, LNA, GLA, or Vitamin F) are found in fats and oils, and are required for the normal function of all of our cells. The term "essential" refers to omega-3 and omega-6 fatty acids, which are not synthesized by the body, and must be obtained from diet. The essential fatty acids (EFAs) are important for the development and function of the brain, neurological, and visual systems. EFAs help prevent stroke and heart disease because they help to reduce cholesterol and triglycerides, while increasing the "good" HDL in the blood profile. EFAs can also help prevent allergies, cancer, menstrual pain, and menopausal hot flashes, and help reduce IBS, ulcerative colitis, migraine headaches, varicose veins, eczema, and psoriasis. Reproductive failure, skin lesions, and behavioral disorders can occur in the absence of the right balance of EFAs. EFAs are also precursors to hormone-like substances called eicosanoids, which regulate many of the vital organ systems in the body. Some research shows a reduction in symptoms associated with lupus, diabetes, and multiple sclerosis. EFAs also help to improve the condition of hair and skin. Because omega-3 fatty acids are natural anti-inflammatory agents, they can help with joint pain, osteoarthritis, rheumatoid arthritis, and gout. Proper doses of Evening Primrose oil have been used to help treat PMS and diabetic neuropathy.

The EFAs we are missing are usually omega-3s. Some people tout fish oil as a good source of omega-3s, but the omega-3s in fish oils are highly unstable molecules that tend to decompose and, in the process, can unleash dangerous free radicals. Some say that this can be counteracted by taking vitamin E, but omega-3s are found in a more stable form in green vegetables and beans, which are also are less expensive than fish (who get their own omega-3s from marine algae).

Americans almost always get too many omega-6 fatty acids (found in grains, certain oils, and processed, fatty foods), and not enough omega-3 fatty acids. Most people can benefit from the switch to an omega-3:omega-6 ratio of 3–4:1. To make the switch, reduce the amount of packaged foods, animal products, trans fats, saturated fats, and omega-6 oils (corn, cottonseed, sunflower, and safflower) in your diet. If you cook with oils, reduce the overall amount and switch to olive or canola oil. Sprinkling ground flax seeds into fruit shakes, salads, hot breakfast cereal, or cold salads is an easy way to get extra omega-3s into your diet. You can also bake with ground flax seeds, or purchase cereals, frozen waffles, or breads made with ground flax seeds. Preventive medicine experts recommend one to two tablespoons of ground flax seeds or an ounce of walnuts each day for those wanting to ensure adequate omega-3 intake. In cases where conversion to DHA may be compromised (e.g., pregnancy, lactation, diabetes), DHA microalgae sources are currently available from Martek and OmegaTech. Leafy green vegetables are not as high in omega-3s as flax or walnuts, but they can also help with EFA balance. Go for variety, and choose whole, fresh, organic produce as often as possible.

Symptoms of Low EFA
Along with the complications listed above, inadequate EFA intake can result in abnormalities of the liver or kidneys, reduced growth rate, impaired fertility, decreased immune function, and dry or scaly skin. Imbalances occur especially in the presence of excess omega-6 and inadequate omega-3.

What Works against EFAs?
Smoking, aging, alcohol, environmental toxins, and excessive saturated fatty acids can inactivate the EFA process in your body. Consuming hard, hydrogenated, and overheated fats will interfere with the vital functions of EFAs. Heating polyunsaturated oils changes the structure of essential fatty acids into toxins called lipid peroxides, which are implicated in cancer and other diseases. Protect flaxseed oil from light, oxygen, and heat by keeping it in its closed container in the refrigerator. Since some prescription and over-the-counter medications will impair your body's ability to

absorb or use nutrients, talk with your doctor about ensuring adequate essential fatty acid intake.

About Supplements
Natural, whole, and unrefined plant food sources are your best bet for overall health and prevention of nutrient deficiency. Whole foods contain vitamins, minerals, fiber, protein, fat, carbohydrate, and phytonutrients in a wonderful variety of balanced combinations. Oils of any kind can increase many disease processes. If you are considering a nutrient supplement or prescription, always work together with your doctor (or with a dietitian) to determine the correct dose. Try to take supplements with a food that contains the nutrient to help your body better absorb and use it. Remember—if you have a kidney, liver, or digestive ailment, or other serious illness, you will need to be especially careful with supplementation.

For more information, contact the Physicians Committee for Responsible Medicine at (202) 686-2210, or at www.pcrm.org. The American Medical Association recommends that you make changes to your current lifestyle

FOOD SOURCES FOR ESSENTIAL FATTY ACIDS

Black currant seeds (Omega-6)	Green beans	Pumpkin
Borage (Omega-6)	Ground flax seeds	Purslane
Broccoli	Honeydew	Radishes
Brussels sprouts	Kale	Romaine lettuce
Cabbage	Kidney beans	Rutabaga
Canola oil	Kohlrabi	Soy beans
Cantaloupe	Leeks	Spinach
Casaba	Lima beans	Tofu
Citrus fruits	Mint	Turnip
Cucumber	Navy beans	Walnuts
Evening Primrose (Omega-6)	Oranges	Watercress
	Peas	Wheat germ
	Perilla	Zucchini
Flaxseed oil	Pinto beans	

regimen with the consultation of your physician. This information is not meant to replace the medical counsel of your doctor or individual consultation with a registered dietitian. Your health care provider and local health department can also be good resources for information on alcohol, tobacco, and other drugs. It is wise to keep yourself educated about health and seek reputable resources when considering changes to your current food and fitness lifestyle.

© Kerrie Saunders, *The Vegan Diet as Chronic Disease Prevention*, New York: Lantern Books, 2003

EXERCISE

A World of Difference

With conveniences like automobiles, appliances, furnaces, plumbing, electricity, outdoor yard equipment, grocers, packaged foods, restaurants, and retail stores, we simply do not get the same amount of exercise through daily living that other generations achieved. All of these conveniences do make daily life easier, but we have sacrificed overall health in many different ways. International research has shown us that cultures that do not rely on "modern conveniences" simply do not have the chronic disease statistics that plague Americans today. A well-planned exercise routine can help give us the best of both worlds: modern conveniences *and* the health to enjoy them more fully.

About Exercise

An overall exercise plan for total fitness should help us maintain strength, stamina, and flexibility. For example, weight training helps build muscle, swimming helps build stamina, and yoga encourages flexibility. Any form of regular, healthy exercise will enhance the immune system, making it easier for the body to prevent and heal illness and injury.

Exercise can be done individually, with family, with a partner, in a class, or as a team with a common goal. Some activities are done indoors, some outdoors, and some can be done in almost any climate. Video instruction can help you learn new exercises and sports, or advance existing skills. For general health maintenance, plan for either three to four one-hour sessions per week, including a 10-minute warmup, 40 minutes of aerobic exercise, and a 10-minute cool-down, or a brisk, daily walk of 30 minutes to one hour. Some people also incorporate "active rest" days in between, where they might enjoy bowling, taking the family to the park, or a low-stress weekly team sport for fun. *The most important thing to remember as you set up your unique routine is to find a variety of activities that you enjoy doing.* Examples of various activities, sports, and exercises are shown in the list below, but feel free to make up your own!

Why Warm Up and Cool Down?

Completing a proper warm-up and cool-down are very important for injury prevention and maximum benefit. The warm-up stimulates blood flow and oxygen to the lungs, muscles and ligaments to prepare them for the work ahead. The cool-down helps to release the lactic acid that has built up in the muscles you just worked, and helps to normalize your heart rate. In this way, the cool-down helps prevent painful injuries, which require time out to heal.

Exercise for Weight Loss

If you are exercising to lose excess weight, a general rule is to plan for four to six one-hour sessions per week. In that hour, you'll have about a 10-minute warm-up, 40 minutes of aerobic exercise, and about a 10-minute cool-down. Aerobic activities increase and sustain your heart rate. Work with your doctor regarding your health and fitness level if you are starting a new routine or advancing to a more athletic level. To break out of the vicious cycle created by inactivity, find the activities you love to do, make a plan, and go for it!

A Quick Note on Steroids and Other Supplements

Anabolic steroids, like those used illegally in sports, are dangerous because they can alter muscle tissue but do not strengthen the ligament, which holds the muscle to the bone. Most "protein" shakes and compounds also contain chemical additives, and can contribute to liver and kidney distress because they often exceed the preventive medicine standards of 10–15% calories from protein. In general, whole and unrefined plant food sources are your best bet for overall health and prevention of nutrient deficiency. Whole foods contain vitamins, minerals, fiber, protein, fat, carbohydrate, and phytonutrients in a wonderful variety of balanced combinations. If you are considering a nutrient supplement or prescription, always work together with your doctor (or with a dietitian) to determine the correct dose. Try to take supplements with a food that contains the nutrient to help your body better absorb and use it. Remember—if you have a kidney, liver, or digestive ailment, or other serious illness, you will need to be especially careful with supplementation.

COMMON FORMS OF EXERCISE

Aerobic dance	Kickboxing	Surfing
Ballet	Martial arts	Swimming
Baseball	Race-walking	Tai Chi
Basketball	Racquetball	Tap dancing
Belly dancing	Rowing	Tennis
Biking	Running	Vigorous yardwork
Breathwork	Scuba diving	Volleyball
Canoeing	Skiing	Walking
Football	Snorkeling	Water polo
Gymnastics	Soccer	Weightlifting
Hiking	Squash	Yoga
Hockey	Stretching	

For more information, contact the Physicians Committee for Responsible Medicine at (202) 686-2210, or at www.pcrm.org. The American Medical Association recommends that you make changes to your current lifestyle regimen with the consultation of your physician. This information is not meant to replace the medical counsel of your doctor or individual consultation with a registered dietitian. Your health care provider and local health department can also be good resources for information on alcohol, tobacco, and other drugs. It is wise to keep yourself educated about health and seek reputable resources when considering changes to your current food and fitness lifestyle.

© Kerrie Saunders, *The Vegan Diet as Chronic Disease Prevention*, New York: Lantern Books, 2003

FIBER

Properties and Benefits

Adequate fiber intake helps provide optimal health and prevent many diseases. Fiber is the structural material of plants, found only in fruits, vegetables, whole grains, beans, nuts, and other seeds. It is a type of carbohydrate that the human body cannot break down. Although it is not digested or metabolized like vitamins and minerals, it serves other important functions. For example, fiber provides a "time release" of vitamins, minerals, fats, and sugars during digestion—helping to optimize the metabolism of these nutrients, and also to prevent blood sugar swings. Fiber provides a feeling of satisfaction, which can help prevent overeating. Fiber also helps the 27 to 30 foot human intestine muscle move waste along, thereby helping to prevent colon cancer.

Two Types of Fiber

Animals and animal products never contain fiber. Both types of fiber, soluble and insoluble, are found only in plant foods—like fruits, vegetables, whole grains, and legumes. We need both soluble and insoluble fiber, and they are each provided in a wonderful balance with the vitamins, minerals, phytonutrients, and antioxidants present in all plant foods.

Soluble fiber helps lower blood cholesterol, especially the plaque-forming LDL cholesterol. Soluble fiber can also help control diabetes, by helping the hormone insulin to work more efficiently. It helps food move into the intestine at a normal rate, which keeps blood sugar from rising rapidly and usually allows diabetes patients to take less medication. Pectin, a type of soluble fiber, binds to fatty substances in the digestive tract, keeping some fat from being absorbed. Common sources of soluble fiber include oats, corn, beans, carrots, peas, lentils, rice bran, barley, citrus fruits, strawberries, and apples. To maximize the benefits of cholesterol-lowering fiber, exercise regularly, and do not smoke.

Insoluble fiber, also called roughage, is a coarse material that does not dissolve in water. It is an important aid to healthy bowel function, because it swells and softens the stool, stimulating the intestinal muscle to move the waste along. This helps to prevent constipation. By moving waste through the colon, insoluble fiber decreases the time that potentially harmful substances in food waste linger in the intestines and come in contact with the intestinal lining. Insoluble fiber also helps with weight control because it binds to water, creating bulk that makes you feel full. Foods that provide insoluble fiber include whole grains, cereals, and breads, wheat bran, rye, rice, barley, seeds, cabbage, beets, carrots, Brussels sprouts, turnips, cauliflower, and the skins of fruits and root vegetables.

How Much Fiber Do I Need?

The healthy adult body needs about 30–35 grams of fiber a day. Unfortunately, most Americans eat less than half the recommended fiber intake per day. A child's daily fiber requirements can be calculated by adding five to the age of the child. For example, a three-year-old child needs 8 grams of fiber each day.

If you're not getting enough fiber, remember that adding whole food sources is better than adding fiber supplements, or relying upon packaged commercial "bran" products such as muffins or waffles, which often contain very little bran. Packaged products may also be high in fat, sugar, and sodium, so read your labels carefully. Processed foods, like enriched breads and crackers, almost always have most of the fiber removed, so reach instead for the whole grain variety. You can also purchase fresh, organic produce to eat raw and unpeeled whenever possible.

Symptoms of Low Fiber Intake

Along with the complications listed above, inadequate fiber intake will usually result in unhealthy bowel movements. A healthy bowel movement should occur about two to three times per day, with no straining, pushing, burning, or bleeding. It should take about as much time to eliminate as the urination. A bowel movement should never hurt, cause hemorrhoids, or lead to bleeding. Diarrhea and constipation are indicators that something is going wrong. Remember, there is no fiber in any animal products.

If you are eating the general recommendation of about 30–35 grams of fiber a day, and you experience constipation or cramping, be certain you are drinking about five to eight glasses of water daily. Adding too much fiber in diet too quickly can cause constipation, diarrhea and bloating, intestinal gas and other digestive discomforts. These side effects usually go away after a short period, especially when you drink adequate amounts of water. Introduce more high-fiber whole foods into your diet gradually to avoid digestive discomfort. If problems persist, see your physician at once.

About Supplements

Natural, whole, and unrefined plant food sources are your best bet for overall health and prevention of nutrient deficiency. Whole foods contain vitamins, minerals, fiber, protein, fat, carbohydrate, and phytonutrients in a wonderful variety of balanced combinations. If you are considering a nutrient supplement or prescription, always work together with your doctor (or with a dietitian) to determine the correct dose. If you do decide to take a fiber supplement, be certain to drink the recommended amount of water. Remember—if you have a kidney, liver, or digestive ailment, or other serious illness, you will need to be especially careful with supplementation.

FOOD SOURCES FOR FIBER

Any fruit
Any vegetable
Any legume (beans, peas, lentils, etc.)
Any whole grain (quinoa, rice, amaranth, wheat, rye, barley, oats, spelt, millet, etc.)
Edible seeds (pumpkin, sesame, sunflower, etc.)

For more information, contact the Physicians Committee for Responsible Medicine at (202) 686-2210, or at www.pcrm.org. The American Medical Association recommends that you make changes to your current lifestyle regimen with the consultation of your physician. This information is not meant to replace the medical counsel of your doctor or individual consultation with a registered dietitian. Your health care provider and local health department can also be good resources for information on alcohol, tobacco, and other drugs. It is wise to keep yourself educated about health and seek reputable resources when considering changes to your current food and fitness lifestyle.

© Kerrie Saunders, *The Vegan Diet as Chronic Disease Prevention*, New York: Lantern Books, 2003

HIGH BLOOD PRESSURE
(Modified from *High Blood Pressure*,
Physicians Committee for Responsible Medicine)

What Is High Blood Pressure?
High blood pressure (hypertension) increases the risk of dangerous health problems, such as heart attacks and strokes. Doctors measure blood pressure using two numbers, such as 120/80. The first number shows the surge of pressure in the arteries with every heart beat, and the second number shows the pressure between beats. If either one of these numbers is too high, blood pressure can be dangerous.[1]

- Optimal   120/80 or less
- Normal   139/89 or less
- Hypertension   140/90 or higher

Imagine a hose (your artery) that now has a build-up of wax (cholesterol) and grease (fat) on its inside walls. Obviously, the flow of fluid (blood) becomes less efficient over time. The human body will then send signals to the brain asking for more blood flow to provide life-giving oxygen and nutrients, so the brain tells the heart to pump harder. If the sludge or blockages are still present in the arteries, the blood and its contents are now pushed harder through smaller openings, like when you squeeze the opening of a garden hose to increase its pressure. This abnormally high fluid pressure can cause ruptures to an already damaged artery wall, causing a heart attack, stroke, or other circulatory problems. Obviously, bringing blood pressure under control is very important. Treatment often involves taking medication, but changing the way you eat can often bring your blood pressure down and reduce the need for medication.

Lifestyle Factors
Health professionals today look to prevent, stop, or reverse many chronic diseases by teaching people to make better choices. Upgrading your diet and exercise can make a world of difference in

your overall health. For example, maintaining a healthy body weight is a common goal in normalizing blood pressure. Avoiding fatty foods such as animal products and fried foods, and increasing the use of whole grains, vegetables, fruits, and beans helps reduce weight and bring down blood pressure. As an added benefit, losing weight reduces your risk of diabetes, heart problems, joint problems, some cancers, and other conditions. If you have a significant weight problem, be sure to consult with your doctor about the best ways for you to lose weight.

Become more physically active. Exercise can also help bring down your blood pressure. A typical healthy exercise schedule would include a brisk walk for a half hour each day or one hour three times per week. Since exercise puts added strain on your heart, be sure to check with your doctor first about the best way for you to become more physically active.

Avoid tobacco. There are many good reasons to quit smoking, and healthier arteries is one of them. Alcohol can raise blood pressure, and it helps to limit alcohol to no more than one to two drinks per day (beer and wine count as drinks). Salt excess can upset potassium balance and increase blood pressure, so follow these tips:

- Use less and less salt in cooking. Your taste will soon adjust.
- Avoid adding salt to foods at the table.
- Avoid salty snacks, such as potato chips.
- Avoid canned foods with added sodium (salt). Choose low-sodium (low-salt) varieties of canned soups and vegetables, or fresh or frozen vegetables, which are naturally low in sodium.
- Read the "Nutrition Facts" label on packaged foods, and be aware of common label claims:
  - Low Sodium—contains 140 mg or less sodium per serving
  - Very Low Sodium—contains 35 mg or less sodium per serving
  - Sodium Free—contains less than 5 mg of sodium per serving

Plant Foods and Blood Pressure

Eat more plant-based (vegetarian) foods. People who follow vegetarian diets typically have lower blood pressure.[2] The American Dietetic Association acknowledges many benefits of a vegetarian diet, including a lower incidence of hypertension when compared to those who eat the Standard American Diet (SAD).[3] No one knows exactly why these foods work so well, but it is probably because cutting out meat, dairy products, and added fats reduces the blood's viscosity (or "thickness"), which, in turn, brings down blood pressure.[4] Plant products are generally lower in fat and sodium and have no cholesterol at all. Vegetables and fruits are also rich in potassium, which helps lower blood pressure.

Try following a vegetarian diet for four to six weeks to find out how well these foods will work for you. Then have your doctor check your blood pressure. Pure vegetarian diets—diets that do not contain any meat, chicken, fish, poultry, eggs, dairy, or animal fat—are generally adequate in all nutrients except vitamin B12, which is found in fortified cereals and high-quality multivitamins. Include more of the following foods in your diet, which are naturally low in sodium:

- **Whole grains**—brown rice, whole wheat bread or pasta, unsweetened hot or cold cereal, millet, barley, buckwheat groats, and quinoa
- **Beans/legumes**—dried (not canned) black-eyed peas, kidney beans, pinto beans, lentils, navy beans, chick peas, soy milk, textured vegetable protein, and tofu
- **Vegetables**—fresh or frozen varieties, such as broccoli, mustard greens, collard greens, kale, spinach, carrots, potatoes, tomatoes, squash, and corn
- **Fruits**—fresh or frozen varieties, such as bananas, oranges, apples, pears, grapefruit, strawberries, mangoes, papayas, guava, strawberries, and blueberries

Let your doctor know you are concerned about your blood pressure and want to use foods to help bring it under control. High blood pressure is dangerous, so, let your doctor guide you as to when and if your need for medication has changed.

References

1. "The sixth report of the Joint National Committee on Prevention, Detection, Evaluation, and Treatment of High Blood Pressure," *Archives of Internal Medicine* 1997; 157: 2413–46.
2. Rouse I. L., Beilin L. J., "Editorial review: vegetarian diet and blood pressure," *Journal of Hypertension* 1984; 2: 231–40.
    Lindahl O., Lindwall L., Spangberg A., Stenram A., Ockerman P. A., "A vegan regimen with reduced medication in the treatment of hypertension," *British Journal of Nutrition* 1984; 52: 11–20.
3. "Position of the American Dietetic Association: Vegetarian Diets," *Journal of the American Dietetic Association* 1997; 97; 11: 1317–21.
4. Ernst E., Pietsch L., Matrai A., Eisenberg J., "Blood rheology in vegetarians," *British Journal of Nutrition* 1986; 56: 555–60.

Authors and Resources

American Dietetic Association Vegetarian Practice Group; Physicians Committee for Responsible Medicine; Charles Attwood, M.D.; Brenda Davis, R.D.; George Eisman, R.D.; Caldwell Esselstyn, M.D.; Joel Fuhrman, M.D.; William Harris, M.D.; Suzanne Havala, M.S., R.D., F.A.D.A.; Michael Klaper, M.D.; Reed Mangels, Ph.D., R.D., F.A.D.A.; John McDougall, M.D.; Vesanto Melina, M.S., R.D.; Dean Ornish, M.D.; Jennifer Raymond, R.D.; Virginia Messina, M.P.H., R.D.; Sharon Yntema, M.A.

For more information, contact the Physicians Committee for Responsible Medicine at (202) 686-2210, or at www.pcrm.org. The American Medical Association recommends that you make changes to your current lifestyle regimen with the consultation of your physician. This information is not meant to replace the medical counsel of your doctor or individual consultation with a registered dietitian. Your health care provider and local health department can also be good resources for information on alcohol, tobacco, and other drugs. It is wise to keep yourself educated about health and seek reputable resources when considering changes to your current food and fitness lifestyle.

IRON

Properties, Benefits, and Healthy Sources

Iron is found in every cell of our body. Most of it is in the hemo-globin of our red blood cells, which is responsible for carrying oxy-gen from our lungs out to the rest of our body. Iron is also needed for normal brain development and the prevention of learning dis-orders in infants and children. Plant foods containing iron are called "non-heme" sources of iron, and, while their iron is not as readily absorbed as the iron in "heme" sources, they do not contain the cholesterol, animal protein, and saturated fat of "heme" iron sources. Legumes and dark green vegetables have more iron per calorie than most meats, and, according to Brenda Davis, R.D., the body uses both forms of iron in the same way. You can increase your body's ability to use "non-heme" iron by eating foods rich in Vitamin C or ascorbic acid. Plant sources of iron include grains, beans, lentils, vegetables, fruits, nuts, and seeds. Go for variety, and choose whole, fresh, organic produce as often as possible.

Symptoms of Low Iron or Anemia

Symptoms of iron-deficiency anemia include paleness, feeling cold, listlessness, fatigue, irritability, difficulty swallowing, muscle weak-ness, heart palpitations during exertion, and lowered resistance to infections. Check with your doctor if you have any of these symp-toms—there are many different forms of anemia, but all types of anemia require attention. Ask your doctor to check for blood loss in stools, which can sometimes be related to an improper, low-fiber diet. According to Dr. John McDougall, a leader in the field of pre-ventive medicine, anemia is actually a sign of an underlying condi-tion producing blood loss, such as bleeding (menstrual, intestinal, trauma), a deficiency of iron, folate, or other B vitamins, excessive blood cell destruction, or a defect in the production of blood cells (like sickle cell anemia, leukemia, rheumatoid arthritis, or kidney failure). It's best to work with your doctor to find out why you are anemic, and correct the problem at its source.

Symptoms of Too Much Iron

Excess iron can cause diarrhea, constipation, abdominal pain, black stools, or indigestion. In cancer patients, it can cause life-threatening incompatibility reactions. Excess iron storage can occur in men—usually from eating a low-fiber diet high in animal and dairy products—and has been associated with an increased risk of heart attack. Too much iron is also associated with the production of free radicals in the blood. Check with your doctor if you have any of these symptoms or concerns.

What Works against Iron?

In addition to the concerns mentioned above, cow milk in infants, caffeine, coffee, tea, antacids, zinc tablets, and oxalates can inhibit the absorption of iron. Phytate, found mainly in whole grains and legumes, can cause poor absorbability of iron, unless the phytate-containing food is leavened, soaked, roasted, or sprouted—or eaten with foods high in vitamin C. Since some prescription and over-the-counter medications will impair your body's ability to absorb or use nutrients, talk with your doctor. For women, a diet high in fats (especially from animal and dairy products) will tend to increase estrogen buildup, which can produce a thicker endometrial tissue inside the uterus, leading to heavier and longer menstrual bleeding. Blood can also be lost in men through ulcers, hemorrhoids, or other abnormalities of the gastrointestinal tract. A well-balanced, plant-based diet contains a safe and adequate amount of iron and helps to prevent such abnormal blood losses.

What Works with Iron?

Cooking with cast-iron pans and eating iron-rich foods with fruit (or citric acid, which is derived from fruit) can help increase your body's access to iron. Ascorbic acid, or vitamin C, will also help with iron absorption and is plentiful in fruits and vegetables. Many whole-grain cereals and pastas or breakfast cereals are fortified with iron, too.

FOOD SOURCES FOR IRON

Almond	Dried fruits	Potatoes
Amaranth	Dulse	Prunes
Artichokes	Enriched oâtmeal	Pumpkin seeds
Arugula	Enriched soy milk	Quinoa
Asparagus	Escarole	Raisins
Avocado	Figs	Red leaf lettuce
Bananas	Garbanzo beans/	Romaine lettuce
Barley	chickpeas	Seeds
Beans	Kale	Sesame seeds
Beets	Kelp	Sorghum
Belgian endive	Kidney beans	Sorrel
Bibb lettuce	Leafy green	Soybeans
Black beans	vegetables	Spinach
Black-eyed peas	Lentils	Sunflower seeds
Bok choy	Lima beans	Swiss chard
Broad beans	Miso	Tofu
Broccoli	Mizuna	Tomatoes
Brown rice	Molasses	Turnip greens
Bulghur wheat	Mustard greens	Wheat germ
Carrots	Nuts	White beans
Cashews	Peanuts	Whole grains
Cherries	Pears	Whole wheat
Chicory	Peas	Whole-grain bagels
Collard greens	Pinto beans	Wild rice
Dandelion greens	Pistachios	

About Supplements

Natural, whole, and unrefined plant food sources are your best bet for overall health and prevention of nutrient deficiency. Whole foods contain vitamins, minerals, fiber, protein, fat, carbohydrates, and phytonutrients in a wonderful variety of balanced combinations. If you or your doctor are considering a nutrient supplement or prescription, always work together (or with a dietitian) to determine the correct dose. If you are pregnant, menstruating, a frequent blood donor, an endurance athlete, or a woman taking hormone replacement therapy, you will want to pay more attention to iron levels, so talk to your doctor. Try to take supplements with a food that contains the nutrient, as a general rule to help your body better absorb and use it. Many dietitians point out that iron and calcium compete for absorption, so it is best to take these supplements at different times. Dietitians advise against iron supplements for individuals with certain disorders, such as hemachromatosis or hemosiderosis. Remember—if you have a kidney, liver, or digestive ailment, or other serious illness, you will need to be especially careful with supplementation.

For more information, contact the Physicians Committee for Responsible Medicine at (202) 686-2210, or at www.pcrm.org. The American Medical Association recommends that you make changes to your current lifestyle regimen with the consultation of your physician. This information is not meant to replace the medical counsel of your doctor or individual consultation with a registered dietitian. Your health care provider and local health department can also be good resources for information on alcohol, tobacco, and other drugs. It is wise to keep yourself educated about health and seek reputable resources when considering changes to your current food and fitness lifestyle.

LACTOSE INTOLERANCE
(or absence of Lactase Persistence)

(Modified from *Understanding Lactose Intolerance*,
Physicians Committee for Responsible Medicine)

What is Lactose Intolerance?

Lactose intolerance is the inability to digest the milk sugar lactose, causing gastrointestinal symptoms of flatulence, bloating, cramps, and diarrhea in some individuals. This results from a shortage of the lactase enzymes that break down lactose into its simpler forms, glucose and galactose, for absorption into the bloodstream. Virtually all infants and young children have these enzymes, and, prior to the mid-1960s, most U.S. health professionals believed that these enzymes were present in nearly all adults as well. When researchers tested various ethnic groups for their ability to digest lactose, however, their findings proved otherwise: Approximately 70% of African Americans, 90% of Asian Americans, 53% of Hispanic Americans, and 74% of Native Americans were lactose intolerant.[1] Studies showed that a substantial reduction in lactase activity is also common among those whose ancestry is Arabic, Jewish, Italian, or Greek.[2]

In 1988, the *American Journal of Clinical Nutrition* reported, "It rapidly became apparent that this pattern was the genetic norm, and that lactase activity was sustained only in a majority of adults whose origins were in Northern European or some Mediterranean populations."[3] In other words, Caucasians tolerate milk sugar only because of an inherited genetic mutation. Overall, about 75% of the world's population, including 25% of those in the United States, lose their lactase enzymes after weaning.[4] The recognition of this fact has resulted in an important change in terminology: Those who could not digest milk were once called "lactose intolerant" or "lactase deficient." They are now regarded as statistically normal, while those adults who retain the enzymes allowing them to digest milk are called "lactase persistent."

There is no reason for people with lactose intolerance to push themselves to drink milk. Indeed, milk and other dairy products do not offer any nutrients that cannot be found in a healthier form in other foods. Surprisingly, drinking milk does not even appear to prevent osteoporosis, though claims to the contrary have been milk's major selling point in recent years.

Milk Does Not Reliably Prevent Osteoporosis

Milk is primarily advocated as a convenient fluid source of calcium in order to slow osteoporosis. However, like the ability to digest lactose, susceptibility to osteoporosis differs dramatically among ethnic groups, and neither milk consumption nor calcium intake in general are decisive factors with regard to bone health. The National Health and Nutrition Examination Survey (NHANES III, 1988–1991) reported that the age-adjusted prevalence of osteoporosis was 21% in U.S. Caucasian women aged 50 years and older, compared with 16% in Hispanic Americans and 10% in African Americans.[5] A 1992 review revealed that fracture rates differ widely among various countries and that calcium intake alone had no clear protective role at all.[6] In fact, those populations with the highest calcium intakes had higher, not lower, fracture rates than those with more modest calcium intakes.

What appears to be important in bone metabolism is not calcium intake alone, but the balance between calcium loss and intake. The loss of bone integrity among many postmenopausal white women probably results from genetics and from diet and lifestyle factors. Research shows that calcium losses are increased by the use of animal protein, salt, caffeine, and tobacco, and by physical inactivity. Animal protein leaches calcium from the bones, leading to its excretion in the urine. Sodium also tends to encourage calcium to pass through the kidneys and is even acknowledged as a contributor to urinary calcium losses in the current *Dietary Guidelines for Americans*.[7] Smoking is yet another contributor to calcium loss. A twin study showed that long-term smokers had a 44% higher risk of bone fracture, compared to a non-smoking identical twin.[8] Physical activity and vitamin D metabolism are also important factors in bone integrity. The balance of these environmental factors, along with genetics, is clearly as important as calcium intake with regard to the risk of osteoporosis and fracture. For most adults worldwide, regular milk consumption can be expected to cause gastrointestinal symptoms, while providing no benefit for the bones.

Commercial Lactase Enzymes: Not the Best Choice

Lactose-reduced commercial milk products are often depicted as the "solution" to lactose intolerance. These products are enzymatically modified to cleave lactose into glucose and galactose, preventing stomach upset and other symptoms of lactose maldigestion. But even with lactase pills and lactose-reduced products, individuals can still experience digestive symptoms. In addition, cow's milk products are low in iron,[9] and a recent study linked cow's milk consumption to chronic constipation in children.[10] Epidemiological studies show a strong correlation between the use of dairy products and the incidence of insulin-dependent diabetes (Type 1 or childhood-onset),[11] and another study showed that women consuming dairy products may have higher rates of infertility and ovarian cancer than those who avoid such products.[12] Susceptibility to cataracts[13] and food allergies are also affected by dairy products.

Healthier Sources of Calcium

While the focus on calcium intake appears to have resulted from the prevalence of osteoporosis among Caucasian women (not to mention the influence of the dairy industry), this is not to say that a certain amount of dietary calcium is not needed by those in other demographic groups. However, calcium is readily available in nondairy sources. Green leafy vegetables, such as broccoli, kale, and collards, are rich in readily absorbable calcium, as shown below.

Many green vegetables have absorption rates of more than 50%, compared with about 32% for milk. In 1994, the *American Journal of Clinical Nutrition* reported calcium absorption to be 52.6% for broccoli, 63.8% for Brussels sprouts, 57.8% for mustard greens, and 51.6% for turnip greens.[14] The calcium absorption rate from kale is approximately 40–59%.[15] Likewise, beans (e.g., pinto beans, black-eyed peas, and navy beans) and bean products, such as calcium-set tofu, are rich in calcium. Also, about 36–38% of the calcium in calcium-fortified orange juice is absorbed (as reported by manufacturer's data).

Green leafy vegetables, beans, calcium-fortified soy milk, and calcium-fortified 100% juices are good calcium sources with advantages that dairy products lack. They are excellent sources of phytochemicals and antioxidants, while containing little fat, no cholesterol, and no animal proteins.

References
1.   Cuatrecasas P., Lockwood D. H., Caldwell J. R., "Lactase deficiency in the adult: a common occurrence," *Lancet* 1965; 1: 14–8.
     Huang S. S., Bayless T. M., "Milk and lactose intolerance in healthy Orientals," *Science* 1968; 160: 83–4.
     Woteki C. E., Weser E., Young E. A., "Lactose malabsorption in Mexican-American adults," *American Journal of Clinical Nutrition* 1977; 30: 470–5.
     Newcomer A. D., Gordon H., Thomas P. J., McGill D. G., "Family studies of lactase deficiency in the American Indian," *Gastroenterology* 1977; 73: 985–8.
2.   Mishkin S., "Dairy sensitivity, lactose malabsorption, and elimination diets in inflammatory bowel disease," *American Journal of Clinical Nutrition* 1997; 65: 564–7.
3.   Scrimshaw N. S., Murray E. B., "The acceptability of milk and milk products in populations with a high prevalence of lactose intolerance," *American Journal of Clinical Nutrition* 1988; 48: 1083–5.
4.   Hertzler S. R., Huynh B. C. L., Savaiano, D. A., "How much lactose is low lactose?" *Journal of the American Dietetic Association* 1996; 96: 243–6.
5.   Looker A. C., Johnston C. C., Wahner H. W., et al., "Prevalence of low femoreal bone density in older U.S. women from NHANES III," *Journal of Bone and Mineral Research* 1995; 10: 796–802.
6.   Abelow B. J., Holford T. R., Insogna K. L., "Cross-cultural association between dietary animal protein and hip fracture: a hypothesis," *Calcified Tissue International* 1992; 50: 14–8.
7.   Nordin B. E. C., Need A. G., Morris H. A., Horowitz M., "The nature and significance of the relationship between urinary sodium and urinary calcium in women," *Journal of Nutrition* 1993; 123: 1615–22.
8.   Hopper J. L., Seeman E., "The bone density of female twins discordant for tobacco use." *New England Journal of Medicine* 1994; 330: 387–92.

FOOD SOURCES OF CALCIUM

Agar	orange juice	Oranges
Almond butter	Carrots	Parsley
Almonds	Chick peas	Pinto beans
Amaranth	Collard greens	Pistachios
Barley	Figs	Raisins
Black turtle beans	Garbanzo beans	Sesame seeds
Blackstrap molasses	Great northern beans	Soybeans
Bok choy	Green beans	Sunflower seeds
Brazil nuts	Hazelnuts	Sweet potatoes
Broccoli	Kale	Tempeh
Brussels sprouts	Kidney beans	Tofu with calcium
Butternut squash	Lentils	Turnip greens
Calcium-fortified	Mustard greens	Vegetarian baked
almond, soy, veg-	Navy beans	beans
gie, or rice milks	Oatmeal	White beans
Calcium-fortified	Okra	Yellow beans

9. Pennington J. A. T., *Bowes and Church's Food Values of Portions Commonly Used*, 17th ed., New York: Lippincott, 1998.
10. Iacono G., Cavataio F., Montalto G., et al., "Intolerance of cow's milk and chronic constipation in children," *New England Journal of Medicine* 1998; 339: 110–4.
11. Scott F. W., "Cow milk and insulin-dependent diabetes mellitus: is there a relationship?" *American Journal of Clinical Nutrition* 1990; 51: 489–91.
    Karjalainen J., Martin J. M., Knip M., et al., "A bovine albumin peptide as a possible trigger of insulin-dependent diabetes mellitus," *New England Journal of Medicine* 1992; 327: 302–7.
12. Cramer D. W., Harlow B. L., Willet W. C., "Galactose consumption and metabolism in relation to the risk of ovarian cancer," *Lancet* 1989; 2· 66–71
13. Simoons F. J., 'A geographic approach to senile cataracts: possible links with milk consumption, lactase activity, and galactose metabolism," *Digestive Disease and Sciences* 1982; 27: 257–64.
14. Weaver C. M., Plawecki K. L., "Dietary calcium: adequacy of a vegetarian diet." *American Journal of Clinical Nutrition* 1994; 59(Suppl): 1238S–41S.
15. Heaney R. P., Weaver C. M., "Calcium absorption from kale," *American Journal of Clinical Nutrition* 1990; 51: 656–7.

For more information, contact the Physicians Committee for Responsible Medicine at (202) 686-2210, or at www.pcrm.org. The American Medical Association recommends that you make changes to your current lifestyle regimen with the consultation of your physician. This information is not meant to replace the medical counsel of your doctor or individual consultation with a registered dietitian. Your health care provider and local health department can also be good resources for information on alcohol, tobacco, and other drugs. It is wise to keep yourself educated about health and seek reputable resources when considering changes to your current food and fitness lifestyle.

© Kerrie Saunders, *The Vegan Diet as Chronic Disease Prevention*, New York: Lantern Books, 2003

PHYTONUTRIENTS AND ANTIOXIDANTS

What is a Phytonutrient?
Phytonutrients, also called phytochemicals, are organic components of plants and promote optimal human health. There are literally thousands of phytonutrients, which may be classified as carotenoids, flavonoids, isoflavones, inositol phosphates, lignans, isothiocyanates and indoles, phenols and cyclic compounds, saponins, sulfides and thiols, and terpenes. In general, phytonutrients enhance immunity and cellular communication, alter estrogen metabolism, metabolize other nutrients, help ward off allergic response, fight cancer and serve as antioxidants, and repair DNA damage from toxins like smoking. We hear a lot about carotenoids, for example, which are found in red, orange, and yellow fruits and vegetables. Carotenoids such as beta-carotene help protect humans against many cancers, heart disease, and age-related macular degeneration. Researchers are constantly finding new benefits of each of the phytonutrient categories, so you are probably hearing more and more about the need to increase the amount of plant foods in your diet.

What is an Antioxidant?
Antioxidants like glutathione, the mineral selenium, vitamins A, C, and E, and other phytonutrients protect us from a build-up of excess free radicals. Free radicals, molecules that damage cells by taking electrons from other molecules, are formed during the metabolism of certain foods, and when we are exposed to radiation, too much sun, or pollutants in our food, water, or air. The free radicals are by-products of oxidation—rather like the formation of rust on metal as it is oxidized. The irritation and damage to cells over time can cause degenerative diseases; arthritis; heart, kidney, and artery problems; cancer; and signs of aging. Antioxidants scavenge the excess free radicals, stopping further damage, and then repair the damage done to healthy cells.

About Supplements

Phytonutrients are only found in plants, so natural, whole, and unrefined plant foods are your best bet for overall health and prevention of nutrient deficiency. Whole foods prevent toxic supplement overdose, and they contain vitamins, minerals, phytonutrients, antioxidants, fiber, protein, fat, and carbohydrate in a wonderful variety of balanced combinations. Go for variety, and choose whole, fresh, raw, and organic produce as often as possible. If you are considering a nutrient supplement or prescription, always work together with your doctor and/or dietitian to determine the correct dose. Try to take supplements with a food that contains the nutrient to help your body better absorb and use it. Remember—if you have a kidney, liver, or digestive ailment, or other serious illness, you will need to be especially careful with supplementation.

For more information, contact the Physicians Committee for Responsible Medicine at (202) 686-2210, or at www.pcrm.org. The American Medical Association recommends that you make changes to your current lifestyle regimen with the consultation of your physician. This information is not meant to replace the medical counsel of your doctor or individual consultation with a registered dietitian. Your health care provider and local health department can also be good resources for information on alcohol, tobacco, and other drugs. It is wise to keep yourself educated about health and seek reputable resources when considering changes to your current food and fitness lifestyle.

© Kerrie Saunders, *The Vegan Diet as Chronic Disease Prevention*, New York: Lantern Books, 2003

FOOD SOURCES OF PHYTONUTRIENTS AND ANTIOXIDANTS

Any fruit

Any vegetable

Any legume (beans, peas, lentils, etc.)

Any whole grain (quinoa, rice, amaranth, wheat, rye, barley, oats, spelt, millet, etc.)

POTASSIUM

Properties, Benefits, and Healthy Sources

Potassium is used in muscle building and contraction, the neutralization of acids, adrenal gland health, water control and waste elimination, fluid balance needed for enzymatic reactions, heart rhythm normalization, blood and tissue alkalinity, vigor, hair, nerve transmission, recuperative power, skin elasticity, conversion of glucose to glycogen (energy storage), and hormone secretion. It also helps your body use calcium, and regulates your blood pressure. Potassium is stored mainly in lean tissues, and is lost as you sweat. Great sources of potassium are generally found in fruits, vegetables, and legumes, like those in the list below. Go for variety, and reach for whole, fresh, organic produce as often as possible.

Symptoms of Low Potassium

Nausea; listlessness; feelings of apprehension; muscle weakness, spasms, or cramps; irregular heartbeat, tachycardia, or heart failure in extreme cases; abnormally high blood pressure; urinary ammonium wasting; impaired glucose tolerance with impaired insulin secretion; impaired protein synthesis; respiratory and vocal cord muscle weakness.

Symptoms of Too Much Potassium

Excess potassium most often occurs in persons with kidney problems, or when potassium supplements are used in an unsafe manner. Signs of toxicity include heart failure, irregular heartbeat, and muscle fatigue.

What Works against Potassium?

Sodium, alcohol, steroids, laxatives, and diuretics all interfere with the absorption or availability of potassium. Fasting, diarrhea, vomiting, prolonged fever, and tissue injury such as surgery or burns can also decrease the bioavailability of potassium. Since some prescription and over-the-counter medications will impair your body's ability to absorb or use nutrients, talk with your doctor.

About Supplements

Natural, whole, and unrefined plant food sources are your best bet for overall health and prevention of nutrient deficiency. Whole foods contain vitamins, minerals, fiber, protein, fat, carbohydrate, and phytonutrients in a wonderful variety of balanced combinations. If you or your doctor is considering a nutrient supplement or prescription, always work together (or with a dietitian) to determine the correct dose. Try to take supplements with a food that contains the nutrient to help your body better absorb and use it. Remember—if you have a kidney, liver, or digestive ailment, or other serious illness, you will need to be especially careful with supplementation.

For more information, contact the Physicians Committee for Responsible Medicine at (202) 686-2210, or at www.pcrm.org. The American Medical Association recommends that you make changes to your current lifestyle reg-

FOOD SOURCES FOR POTASSIUM

Almonds	Cucumber	Parsley	Soybeans
Apple	Currants	Peaches	Spinach
Apricot	Daikon	Peanuts	Spirulina
Arugula	Dates	Pears	Sprouted grains
Avocado	Dulse	Peas	Sprouts
Banana	Figs	Pecans	Squash
Beans	Green cabbage	Pineapple	Sunflower
Beet greens	Kelp	Pistachios	seeds
Broccoli	Legumes	Potato	Sweet potato
Cantaloupe	Lentils	Prunes	Swiss chard
Carrots	Lima beans	Pumpkin	Tomato
Cauliflower	Mango	Pumpkin seeds	Turnip
Celery	Molasses	Radicchio	Watercress
Cherries	Mung beans	Radishes	Wheatgrass
Cilantro	Mushrooms	Raisins	Whole grains
Citrus fruit	Mustard greens	Red cabbage	
Collard greens	Oranges	Rutabaga	
Cranberries	Papaya	Sesame seeds	

imen with the consultation of your physician. This information is not meant to replace the medical counsel of your doctor or individual consultation with a registered dietitian. Your health care provider and local health department can also be good resources for information on alcohol, tobacco, and other drugs. It is wise to keep yourself educated about health and seek reputable resources when considering changes to your current food and fitness lifestyle. © Kerrie Saunders, *The Vegan Diet as Chronic Disease Prevention*, New York: Lantern Books, 2003

PURINES AND GOUT

When Purines Are a Problem

Gout is a form of arthritis, characterized by an excess of uric acid in the blood. The uric acid forms crystal-like deposits, almost like bits of broken glass, which float in the space between the joints. When the immune system tries to attack the crystals (most commonly in the big toe), pain and swelling occur. Although gout is considered hereditary, being overweight and eating too many purine-containing foods can speed up the onset of the disease. Kidney stones are also related to gout conditions.

Getting Gout under Control

While the symptoms of gout can sometimes be managed by prescriptions, a change in your diet and lifestyle can be a great help, maybe even eliminating the need for medication. Among the culprits in gout, we find certain drugs, alcohol, and improper diet. Some authors also implicate excess supplementation with niacin or vitamin A.

FOOD SOURCES TO CONSIDER
AS TRIGGERS FOR GOUT

Animal flesh and organs (beef, pork, bacon, lamb, fish, shellfish, liver, brain, chicken, turkey, eel, venison, etc.)

Animal fluids (cow milk, butter, cheese, cottage cheese, ice cream, meat extracts, goat milk, etc.)

Asparagus

Cauliflower

Legumes (kidney beans, navy and lima beans, lentils, peas)

Mushrooms

Oatmeal

Spinach

Whole grain cereals or breads

Whole wheat germ and bran

Yeast

Be sure to drink at least five glasses of water daily, learn to manage stress, and avoid foods that are high in purines. Foods with a high purine content are listed below, but it may be easier to remember to follow a low-fat, high-fiber vegetarian diet. This diet automatically eliminates most of the major offenders that exacerbate gout—like animal flesh and organs (meat, poultry, venison, brain, tongue, etc.), fish, fish eggs, and shellfish—many of which also contain large amounts of dietary cholesterol and saturated fat. Work with your doctor and/or dietitian based on your body's response to various foods. Doctors and dietitians trained in elimination diets can be of particular help. Learning to avoid your particular trigger foods can make a significant difference in the amount of pain you experience.

More Information on the Optimal Diet for Disease Prevention

Eating for maximum disease prevention means increasing the vitamins, minerals, fiber, antioxidants, and phytonutrients in your diet, while reducing the hormones, antibiotics, cholesterol, saturated fat, excess protein, and concentrated pesticide content normally found in the Standard American Diet. Many physicians and dietitians are now aware of the benefits of proper lifestyle, exercise, and nutrition. The Physicians Committee for Responsible Medicine, Dean Ornish, M.D., Brenda Davis, R.D., Vesanto Melina, R.D., John McDougall, M.D., Joel Fuhrman, M.D., William Harris, M.D., and Michael Klaper, M.D., are all wonderful resources for the health benefits of a low-fat, high-fiber vegetarian diet. Work with your doctor and enjoy your new health!

For more information, contact the Physicians Committee for Responsible Medicine at (202) 686-2210, or at www.pcrm.org. The American Medical Association recommends that you make changes to your current lifestyle regimen with the consultation of your physician. This information is not meant to replace the medical counsel of your doctor or individual consultation with a registered dietitian. Your health care provider and local health department can also be good resources for information on alcohol, tobacco, and other drugs. It is wise to keep yourself educated about health and seek reputable resources when considering changes to your current food and fitness lifestyle.
© Kerrie Saunders, *The Vegan Diet as Chronic Disease Prevention*, New York: Lantern Books, 2003

2/06   9   1/06
5/12   (39)   1/12
3/13   (44)   11/12
9/15   (58) 4/15
2/17   (59)   7/16